FROM BIRTH TO FIVE YEARS

FROM BIRTH TO FIVE YEARS

Children's developmental progress

Mary D. Sheridan

Revised and updated by
Ajay Sharma and Helen Cockerill

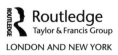
Routledge
Taylor & Francis Group

LONDON AND NEW YORK

First published by the NFER Publishing Company Ltd, 1973
Second impression 1974
Third and expanded edition 1975
Fourth impression 1976
Fifth impression 1977
Sixth impression 1978
Seventh impression 1980

Reprinted by the NFER-Nelson Publishing Company Ltd,
1981, 1982, 1983, 1984, 1985, 1986, 1987, 1988 (twice), 1989, 1990, 1991

Reprinted in 1992 (twice), 1993, 1994 (twice), 1995 by Routledge
2 Park Square, Milton Park, Abingdon, Oxon, OX14 4RN

Revised and updated edition published 1997 by Routledge.

Reprinted 1999, 2000, 2001, 2003, 2004, 2005 (twice)

This revised and updated edition published 2008 by Routledge

Simultaneously published in the USA and Canada
by Routledge
270 Madison Avenue, New York, NY 10016

Reprinted 2009

Routledge is an imprint of the Taylor & Francis Group, an informa business

© 2008 Mary Sheridan; Revised and updated by Ajay Sharma and Helen Cockerill

Typeset in Univers by
Keystroke, 28 High Street, Tettenhall, Wolverhampton
Printed and bound in Great Britain by
TJ International Ltd, Padstow, Cornwall

British Library Cataloguing in Publication Data
A catalogue record for this book is available from the British Library

Library of Congress Cataloging in Publication Data
Sheridan, Mary D. (Mary Dorothy)
    From birth to five years : children's developmental progress / Mary D.
    Sheridan. — 3rd ed. / rev. and updated by Ajay Sharma and Helen Cockerill.
       p. ; cm.
    Includes bibliographical references.
    ISBN 978-0-415-42365-6 (pbk.)
    1. Children—Growth. 2. Child development. I. Sharma, Ajay.
    II. Cockerill, Helen. III. Title.
    [DNLM: 1. Child Development. 2. Child, Preschool. WS 105 S552f 2008]
    RJ131.S5 2008
    618.92—dc22   2007041888

ISBN10: 0–415–42365–1
ISBN13: 978–0–415–42365–6

Contents

Introduction

This revised edition of *From Birth to Five Years* aims to provide concise and clear information on children's developmental progress as a reference source for students and professionals from a wide range of health, education and social-care sectors.

The original edition of this book, based on research carried out by Mary D. Sheridan, was primarily concerned with describing appropriate developmental norms and testing procedures to help in the diagnosis of developmental disorders. Whilst continuing to recognise the importance of detecting disorders and providing effective support for children with special needs, this edition aims to contribute to the development of a common core of skills and knowledge for everyone working with children. This is in line with the current ethos of improving health, educational and social outcomes for all children enshrined in 'Every Child Matters'.

The 'Illustrated Charts of Children's Developmental Progress' in Section 1 are organised into the domains of posture and large movements; visual perceptual and fine motor; hearing; speech, language and communication; social behaviour and play; and self-care and independence. The content of the charts has been updated, with increased emphasis on social communication and perception. These can provide a starting point for eliciting age-appropriate information from parents and carers, for making observations in natural and clinic settings and for obtaining a comparative view of the child's achievements against the average expected achievement: i.e., typical developmental progress.

Section 2, 'Assessing Children's Developmental Progress', provides information and guidance on the sequence of development and key stages within each domain. These chapters discuss factors influencing children's development, the interaction of child-related and context-related factors and markers that help differentiate developmental vulnerability from the wide spectrum of typical development. Practical guidance on eliciting concerns and assessing development and general guidance on facilitating development is provided. New sections on attention, self-regulation, attachment, emotional development and the development of self are provided as an acknowledgement of their significance in children's educational and social outcomes.

The Internet has opened a new world of resources for carers and professionals. An annotated list of web-based resources is provided in addition to 'Further Reading' for each developmental domain.

Illustrated charts of children's developmental progress | Section 1

During the first few days of life, there is a great variability in the behaviour of babies depending not only upon the baby's maturity and physical condition but also upon its state of alertness or drowsiness, hunger or satiation. An examination of the newborn baby must include a discussion with the parents regarding any concerns they have about the behaviour of their newborn baby.

THE NEWBORN BABY

■ The first few days of a baby's life are usually composed of long periods of sleep interspersed with short periods when the baby is awake.

The state of sleep and wakefulness

■ The duration of wakefulness lengthens gradually and includes periods of fretfulness, crying and calmness.

■ The responsiveness of the baby depends on the state of sleep or wakefulness (Brazelton and Nugent 1995).

■ Any examination of the newborn should be carried out in the optimal state of active wakefulness, when the infant is quiet, with eyes open, regular breathing, active limb movements and no crying (Prechtl 1977).

■ At birth, the arms and legs are characteristically stiff (hypertonia) and the trunk and neck floppy (hypotonia).

Posture and large movements

■ Lying on the back (supine), the arms and legs are kept semi-flexed and the posture is symmetrical.

■ Babies born after breech presentation usually keep their legs extended.

■ Pulled to sitting, marked head lag is present.

■ Held in a sitting position, the back is curved, and the head falls forward.

■ Held in ventral suspension, the head drops below the plane of the body, and the arms and legs are kept partly flexed.

■ Placed on the abdomen (prone), the head is promptly turned sideways. The buttocks are humped up, with the knees tucked under the abdomen. The arms are close to the chest with the elbows fully flexed.

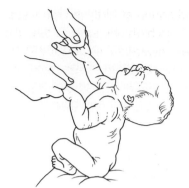
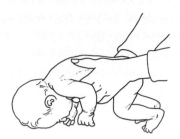

pulled to sit   *ventral suspension*

The primary reflexes

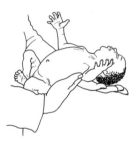

moro reflex

■ These represent neurological maturation of the newborn, and most develop before birth. Some reflexes may help in establishing symmetry of movement, but others are of limited value in the examination of a full-term newborn infant. The Moro reflex is the best-known of all the neonatal reflexes. It can be produced in several ways. The usual method is by sudden, slight (2.5 centimetres) dropping of the examiner's hand supporting the baby's head. The response consists of symmetrical wide abduction of the arms and opening of the hands. Within moments, the arms come together again, simulating an embrace. The reflex fades rapidly and is not normally present after 6 months of age.

■ Reflex rooting and sucking behaviour is apparent unless the baby has just been fed. Infants show nutritive sucking for feeding and non-nutritive sucking patterns (self-calming on fingers or dummies). Rooting fades by 6 months and involuntary suckling by 12 months.

■ Protective gag and cough reflexes are also present, and these persist throughout life.

■ Strong and symmetrical palmar grasp reflex is present but fades rapidly over the next 4 to 5 months.

■ Reflex standing and reflex walking are apparent during the early weeks of life if the feet are placed on a firm surface.

- Babies are sensitive to light and sound at birth though visual responsiveness varies at birth. From birth onwards, or within a few days, infants turn their eyes towards a large and diffuse source of light and close their eyes to sudden bright light. An object or face must be brought to a distance of 30 centimetres to obtain interest and fixation. Infants usually turn their eyes to slowly follow a face.

- The startle reaction to sudden loud sounds is present. Eyes may be turned towards a nearby source of continued sound, such as a voiced 'ah-ah' or a bell. Momentary stilling to weaker, continuous sounds is also seen.

Hearing and vision

- Within a few days of birth, infants establish interaction with their carers through eye contact, spontaneous or imitative facial gestures and modulation of their sleep–wakefulness state.

- Patterns of interaction and subtle indications of individuality shown by babies from birth onwards strengthen the emotional ties between infants and their carers.

Social interaction and formation of attachments

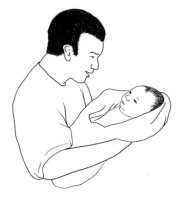

social interaction

AGE 1 MONTH

Posture and large movements

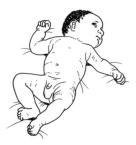

lying on back supine (showing asymmetric tonic neck reflex)

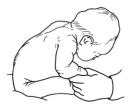

pulled to sit

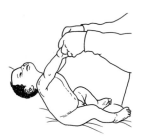

held sitting

■ Lying on back (supine), keeps head to one side. Moves arms and legs in large, jerky movements. At rest, keeps hands closed and thumbs turned in, but beginning to open hands from time to time. Fingers and toes fan out during extensor movements of limbs.

■ When cheek touched at corner of mouth, turns to same side in attempt to suck finger. Pulled to sit, head lags unless supported. Held in supported sitting, head is vertical momentarily before falling forwards, and back is one complete curve.

■ In ventral suspension, holds head in line with body and hips are semi-extended.

■ Placed on abdomen (prone), head immediately turns to side; arms and legs flexed, elbows away from body, buttocks moderately high.

■ Held standing on hard surface, presses down feet, straightens body and usually makes a reflex forward 'walking' movement. Stimulation of dorsum of foot against table edge produces 'stepping up over curb' reflex.

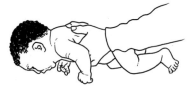

ventral suspension

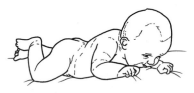

attempts to lift head in prone

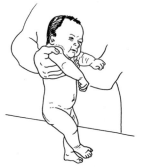

reflex 'walking' movement

- Pupils react to light. Turns head and eyes towards diffuse light source – stares at diffuse brightness of window, table lamp or lightly coloured blank wall.

- Follows pencil light briefly with eyes, at a distance of 30 centimetres. Shuts eyes tightly when pencil light shone directly into them.

- Gaze caught and held by dangling bright toy gently moved in line of vision at 15 to 25 centimetres, towards and away from face. From about 3 weeks, watches familiar nearby face when being fed or talked to with increasingly alert facial expression. Focuses and follows, with eyes, slow movements of face or object from side towards midline horizontally, with some accompanying head movement through quarter circle or more, before head falls back to side.

- Defensive blink present by 6 to 8 weeks.

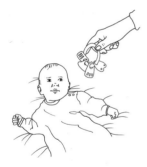

gazes at toy moved towards and away from face

regards familiar face when being fed

turns to diffuse light source

- Startled by sudden noises, stiffens, quivers, blinks, screws up eyes, extends limbs, fans out fingers and toes and may cry.

- Movements momentarily 'frozen' when small bell rung gently; may move eyes and head towards sound source, but cannot yet localise sound.

Hearing behaviour

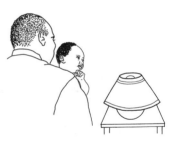

stops whimpering to listen to sudden noise

Speech, language and communication

- Stops whimpering; and usually turns towards sound of nearby soothing human voice or loud and prolonged noise, e.g., vacuum cleaner, but not when screaming or feeding.

- Utters little guttural noises when content.

- Babies have a preference for social stimuli and will coo and make pre-speech lip and tongue movements responsively to parent's or carer's talk from soon after birth.

- Cries lustily when hungry or uncomfortable.

Note: babies with hearing impairment also cry and vocalise in this reflex fashion but when very severely impaired do not usually show startle reflex to sudden noise. Babies with severe visual impairment may also move eyes towards a sound-making instrument. Visual following and auditory response must, therefore, always be tested separately.

Social behaviour and play

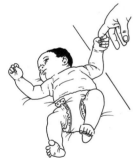

grasps finger

- Sucks well.

- Sleeps most of the time when not being fed or handled.

- Expression still vague but becoming more alert, progressing to social smile and responsive vocalisations at about 5 or 6 weeks.

- Eye-to-eye contact is deliberately maintained or terminated by the infant during social interaction.

- Hands normally closed, but if opened, grasps finger when palm is touched.

- Stops crying when picked up and spoken to. Turns to regard nearby speaker's face.

- Needs support to head when being carried, dressed and bathed.

Self-care and independence

- Passive acceptance of bath and dressing routines gradually gives way to emerging awareness and responsiveness.

- Lying on back, prefers to lie with head in midline. Limbs more pliable, movements smoother and more continuous. Waves arms symmetrically. Hands loosely open.

- Brings hands together in midline over chest or chin. Kicks vigorously, legs alternating or occasionally together.

- When pulled to sit, little or no head lag. Held sitting, back is straight except in lumbar region. Head held erect and steady for several seconds before bobbing forwards.

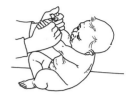

pulled to sit

- In ventral suspension, head held well above line of body, hips and shoulders extended.

- Needs support at shoulders when being bathed and dressed.

- Lying on abdomen, lifts head and upper chest well up in midline, using forearms to support and often actively scratching at surface with hands, with buttocks flat.

- Held standing with feet on hard surface, sags at knees.

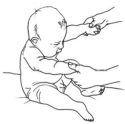

held sitting, with curved back

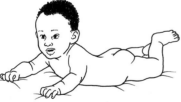

lifts head and shoulders in prone

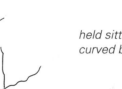

ventral suspension

Visual perceptual and fine motor

- Visually very alert, particularly preoccupied by nearby human face. Moves head deliberately to gaze attentively around. Follows adult's movements within available visual field.

- Follows dangling toy at 15–25 centimetres from face through half circle horizontally from side to side and usually also vertically from chest to brow. Defensive blink is clearly shown.

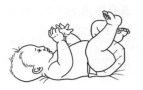

hand regard and finger play

■ Hand regard when lying supine – watches movement of own hands before face and engages in finger play, opening and closing hands and pressing palms of hands together.

■ Regards small still objects within 15–25 centimetres for more than a second or two, but seldom fixates continuously.

■ Converges eyes as dangling toy is moved towards face.

■ Reaches out to grasp with both hands by 16–18 weeks of age.

■ Holds rattle for a few moments when placed in hand, may move towards face – sometimes bashing chin – but seldom capable of regarding it at the same time until 16–18 weeks of age.

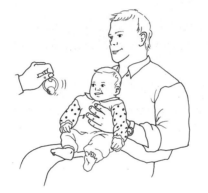

follows dangling toy

holds toy but cannot yet co-ordinate hands and eyes

Hearing behaviour

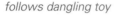

turns to nearby voice

■ Turns eyes and/or head towards sound source, e.g., nearby voice; brows may wrinkle and eyes dilate.

■ May move head from side to side as if searching for sound source.

■ Quietens to sound of rattle or small bell rung gently out of sight.

■ Definite quieting or smiling to sound of familiar voice before being touched, but not when screaming.

Note: babies with severe hearing impairment may be obviously startled by carer's appearance beside cot.

- Cries when uncomfortable or annoyed.

- Often sucks or licks lips in response to sounds of preparation for feeding.

- Shows excitement at sound of approaching voices, footsteps, running bathwater, etc.

- Vocalises delightedly when spoken to or pleased; also when alone. Vocalisations are integrated with smiles, eye contact and hand gestures during turn-taking exchanges or 'protoconversations'.

- Fixes eyes unblinkingly on parent's or carer's face when feeding, with contented purposeful gaze.

- Eager anticipation of breast or bottle feed. Beginning to show reactions to familiar situations by smiling, cooing and excited movements.

- Now definitely enjoys bathing and caring routines. Responds with obvious pleasure to friendly handling, especially when accompanied by playful tickling, child-friendly speech and singing.

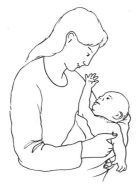

responds with pleasure to friendly handling

AGE 6 MONTHS

Posture and large movements

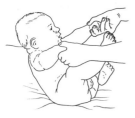

pulls self to sitting, braces shoulders

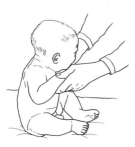

held sitting, back straight

■ Lying on back, raises head up and moves arms up to be lifted.

■ When hands grasped, braces shoulders and pulls self to sitting.

■ Sits with support with head and back straight and turns head from side to side to look around. (Independent sitting without support is achieved from 5 to 9 months.)

■ Can roll over from front to back (prone to supine) at around 5–6 months and usually from back to front (supine to prone) a little later at around 6–7 months (Bly 1994).

■ Placed on abdomen, lifts head and chest well up, supporting self on extended arms and flattened palms.

■ Bears weight on feet and bounces up and down actively when held in supported standing with feet touching hard surface. Protective reflexes begin to appear (see table).

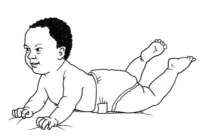

lying on abdomen, arms extended

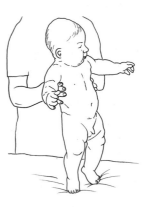

held standing, takes weight on legs

Protective reflexes
These reflexes develop from 4 to 5 months onwards and can be absent or abnormal in motor disorders.

Downward parachute reflex	5 months	When held and rapidly lowered the infant extends and abducts both legs and feet are plantigrade.
Sideward protective reflex	6 months	Infant puts arms out to save if tilted off balance.
Forward protective reflex	7 months	Arms and hands extend on forward descent to ground.
Backward protective reflex	9 months	Backward protective extension of both arms when pushed backwards in sitting position.

(Milani-Comparetti and Gidoni 1967)

Visual perceptual and fine motor development

- Visually insatiable: moves head and eyes eagerly in every direction when attention is distracted. Eyes move in unison. Follows adult's or child's activities across room with purposeful alertness. Immediately stares at interesting small objects or toys within 15–30 centimetres. Shows awareness of depth.

- Stretches out both hands simultaneously to grasp. Uses hands competently to reach for and grasp small toys. Mainly uses two-handed scooping-in approach, but will occasionally use a single hand. Adjusts arm and hand posture to orientation of the object. Uses whole hand to palmar grasp and passes toy from one hand to another. Drops one object if another is offered.

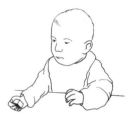

palmar grasp

- When toy falls from hand within visual field, watches to resting place. When toy falls outside visual field, searches vaguely around with eyes and hands, or forgets it (early permanence of object).

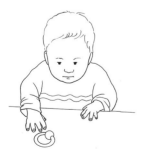

reaches for toy with one hand . . .

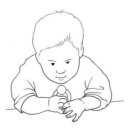

manipulates toy with both hands

Hearing behaviour	■ Turns immediately to a familiar voice across the room.

Hearing behaviour

■ Turns immediately to a familiar voice across the room.

■ Listens to voice even if adult not in view.

■ Turns to source when hears sounds at ear level.

Speech, language and communication

■ Vocalises tunefully to self and others, using sing-song vowel sounds or single and double syllables, e.g., 'a-a', 'muh', 'goo', 'der', 'adah', 'er-leh', 'aroo'.

■ Laughs, chuckles and squeals aloud in play. Screams with annoyance.

■ Shows recognition of carer's facial expressions such as *happy* or *fearful* and responds selectively to emotional tones of voice.

Social behaviour and play

■ Shows delighted response to rough-and-tumble play. Reacts enthusiastically to often-repeated games. Shows anticipation responses if carer pauses before high points in nursery rhymes and other action songs.

■ When offered a rattle, reaches for it immediately and shakes deliberately to make a sound, often regarding it closely at the same time. Manipulates objects attentively, passing them frequently from hand to hand. Takes everything to mouth. When totally absorbed in exploration of objects, may seem oblivious to carer's attempts to engage in interaction.

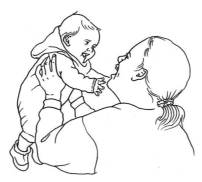

shows delighted response to rough-and-tumble play

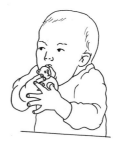

takes everything to mouth

■ Still friendly with strangers but occasionally shows some shyness or even slight anxiety when approached too nearly or abruptly, especially if familiar adult is out of sight. Becomes more reserved with strangers from about 7 months.

■ Places hand on breast while feeding; or if fed with formula milk, puts hand on bottle and pats it. May attempt to grasp cup if used.

Self-care and independence

■ Beginning to take smooth semi-solids. Initially spits out food using back-and-forth tongue movements. Gradually learns to suck food from spoon.

AGE 9 MONTHS

Posture and large movements

- Pulls self to sitting position. Sits unsupported on the floor and can adjust body posture when leaning forward to pick up and manipulate a toy without losing balance.

- Can turn body to look sideways while stretching out to pick up toy from floor.

- Progresses on floor by rolling, wriggling on abdomen or crawling.

- Pulls to standing, holding on to support for a few moments but cannot lower self and falls backwards with a bump.

- Held standing, steps purposefully on alternate feet.

- Only needs intermittent support when sitting on parent's or carer's lap and being dressed. When being carried by an adult, supports self in upright position and turns head to look around.

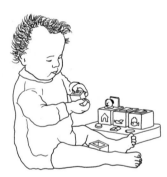
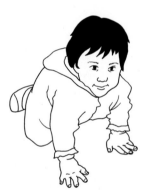
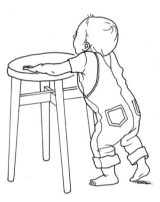

sits on floor and manipulates toys

attempts to crawl

pulls to standing

Visual-perceptual and fine motor

- Visually very attentive to people, objects and happenings in the environment.

- Most fundamental visual functions, such as depth perception for working out the relative position of objects in visual field and smooth visual attention to moving objects, are now in place.

- Immediately stretches out to grasp a small toy when offered, with one hand leading. Manipulates toy with a lively interest, passing from hand to hand and turning over.

- Regards unoffered but accessible toy before grasping, especially if unfamiliar.

- Can reach and grasp a moving object by moving towards the anticipated position of the moving object.

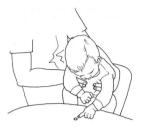

pokes at small objects using index finger

- Pokes at small object with index finger and begins to point at more distant object with same finger.

- Grasps string between finger and thumb in scissor fashion in order to pull toy towards self.

- Picks up small object between finger and thumb with 'inferior' pincer grasp.

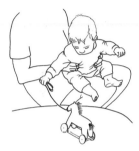

grasps string to pull toy

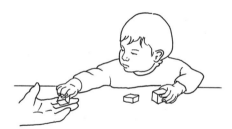

attempts to give block, but cannot yet release

picks up small object with pincer grasp

- Can release toy from grasp by dropping or pressing against a firm surface but cannot yet release smoothly.

- Enjoys casting objects over the side of cot or chair.

- Looks in correct direction for falling or fallen toys (permanence of object).

- Shows understanding of things that are causally connected, e.g., plays with cause-and-effect toys and pulls on a string to get the connected toy (causal understanding).

■ Watches activities of people or animals within 3 or 4 metres with sustained interest for several minutes.

Hearing behaviour

■ Eagerly attentive to everyday sounds, particularly voice.

■ Turns to search and localise faint sounds on either side.

■ Locates sounds made above and below ear level.

Speech, language and communication

■ Vocalises deliberately as a means of interpersonal communication in friendliness or annoyance. Shouts to attract attention, listens, then shouts again.

■ Babbles loudly and tunefully in long repetitive strings of syllables, e.g., 'dad-dad', 'mum-mum', 'adaba', 'agaga'. Babble is practised largely for self-amusement, but also within 'conversations' with carers.

■ Responds when name is called (Fenson et al. 1993).

■ Understands 'no' and 'bye-bye'.

■ Reacts to 'where's mummy/daddy?' by looking around.

■ Imitates playful vocal and other sounds, e.g., smacking lips, cough, 'brrr'.

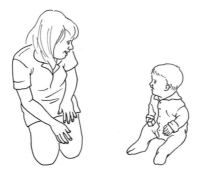

turns to sound, such as when name is called

Note: The vocalisations of children with severely impaired hearing remain at the primitive level and do not usually progress to repetitive tuneful babble. Poor or monotonous vocalisations after 8 or 9 months of age should always arouse suspicion.

- Throws body back and stiffens in annoyance or resistance, usually protesting vocally at same time.

- Clearly distinguishes strangers from familiars and requires reassurance before accepting their advances; clings to known person and hides face.

- Still takes everything to mouth.

- Grasps bell by handle and rings in imitation. Shakes a rattle, explores it with a finger and bangs on floor.

- Plays 'peek-a-boo' and imitates hand-clapping.

- Offers food to familiar people and animals.

- Grasps toy in hand and offers to adult but cannot yet give into adult's hand.

- Watches toy being partially hidden under a cover or cup, and then finds it. May find toy wholly hidden under cushion or cup.

- Sustained interest for up to full minute in looking at pictures named by adult.

Social behaviour and play

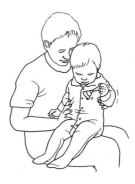

grasps bell by hands and rings in imitation

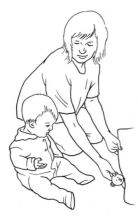
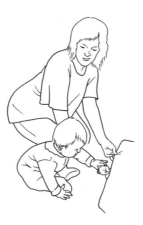

watches while toy is partly hidden . . .   *. . . and promptly finds toy*

**Self-care and
independence**

■ Holds, bites and chews a small piece of food.

■ Puts hands on breast or around bottle or cup when drinking.

■ Tries to grasp spoon when being fed.

■ Enjoys babbling with a mouthful of food.

- Sits on floor for indefinite time. Can rise to sitting position from lying down with ease.

- Crawls on hands and knees, shuffles on buttocks or 'bearwalks' rapidly about the floor. May crawl upstairs.

- Pulls to standing and sits down again, holding onto furniture. Walks around furniture lifting one foot and stepping sideways. May stand alone for a few moments.

- Walks forwards and sideways with one or both hands held. May walk alone.

AGE 12 MONTHS

Posture and large movements

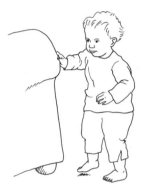 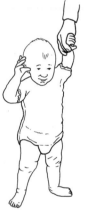

bearwalks around floor   *cruises, holding onto furniture*   *walks with one hand held*

- Out of doors, watches movement of people, animals or motor vehicles for prolonged periods. Recognises familiar people approaching from a distance. Shows interest in pictures.

- Has a mature grasp. Picks up small objects with neat pincer grasp between thumb and tip of index finger. By 13 months, reaching and grasping become coordinated into one smooth action, e.g., closing of hand starts during approach and well before touching the object.

- Drops and throws toys forwards deliberately and watches them fall to ground. Looks in correct place for toys which fall out of sight.

Visual perceptual and fine motor

■ Points with index finger at objects of interest.

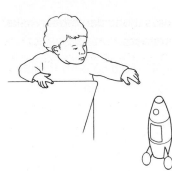

*points with index finger
to objects of interest*

■ Uses both hands freely but may show preference for one. Holds two toy bricks, one in each hand with tripod grasp, and bangs together to make noise.

Hearing behaviour

■ Locates sounds from any direction well. Immediately responds to own name.

■ Shows recognition of familiar tunes by trying to join in.

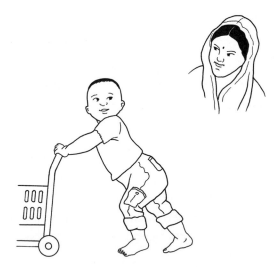

immediately responds to own name

- Babbles loudly and incessantly in conversational cadences (jargon). Vocalisation contains most vowels and many consonants.

- Shows by behaviour that some words are understood in usual context, e.g., car, drink, cat. Understands simple instructions associated with a gesture, e.g., 'Give it to Daddy', 'Come to Mummy'.

- Frequently responds to familiar songs by vocalising. Imitates adult playful vocalisations e.g., 'uh-oh' and may use a few words.

- Will follow the gaze of an adult (joint visual attention). Points to objects and then looks back to the adult for a reaction, for the purposes of requesting or eliciting a comment from the adult (Tomasello 1995).

Speech, language and communication

- Takes objects to mouth less often. Very little, if any, drooling of saliva.

- Will put objects in and out of cup or box when shown.

- Likes to be in sight and hearing of familiar people. Demonstrates affection to familiars.

- Plays 'pat-a-cake' and waves 'good-bye', both on request and spontaneously.

- Enjoys joint play with adults, actively switching attention between objects and adult (co-ordinated joint attention).

Social behaviour and play

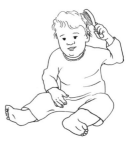

understanding-by-use of everyday objects

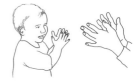

plays 'pat-a-cake'

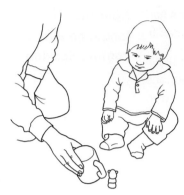
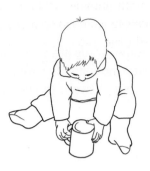
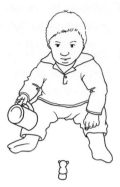

watches while toy is hidden under cup

lifts cup to search for the toy

promptly finds toy, and looks to adult

- Manipulates toys and will shake to make noise. Listens with pleasure to sound-making toys and repeats appropriate activity to reproduce sound.

- Gives toys to adults on request and sometimes spontaneously.

- Demonstrates understanding by use of objects, e.g., hair brush (definition-by-use).

- Quickly finds toys hidden from view.

Self-care and independence

- Drinks well from cup with little assistance.

- Holds spoon and will attempt to use for feeding, although very messy.

- Munches chopped food at sides of mouth.

- Sits, or sometimes stands, without support while dressed by carer.

- Helps with dressing by holding out arm for sleeve and foot for shoe.

- May walk alone, usually with uneven steps: feet wide apart, arms slightly flexed and held above head or at shoulder level for balance. Walks with broad base, high stepping gait and steps of unequal length. Starts voluntarily but frequently stopped by falling or bumping into furniture.

  Note: infants who 'bottom shuffle' are usually delayed in walking.

- Lets self down from standing to sitting by collapsing backward with a bump, or by falling forwards on hands and then back to sitting. Can get back to feet alone.

- Creeps upstairs safely and may get downstairs backwards.

- Kneels unaided or with support.

- Watches small toy pulled across floor. Demands desired objects out of reach by pointing with index finger. Stands at window and watches outside happenings with interest. Attends to coloured pictures in book and pats page.

- Picks up string or small objects with a precise pincer grasp, using either hand.

- Manipulates cubes and may build a tower of two cubes after demonstration. Can take objects out of container and replace fairly precisely, e.g., pegs in holes.

- Grasps crayon with whole hand, using palmar grasp. Uses either hand and imitates to-and-fro scribble.

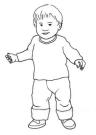
Visual perceptual and fine motor

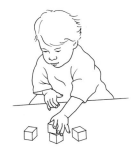

manipulates blocks and builds tower of two

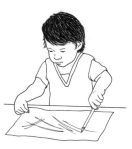

grasps crayon with whole hand and scribbles to and fro

Speech, language and communication

- Makes many speech-like sounds.

- Says a few recognisable words (usually a range of between two to six) spontaneously in correct context and demonstrates understanding of many more.

- Appears to understand some new words each week.

- Will sustain interest for two or more minutes in looking at pictures in a book if they are named (Bzoch and League 1991).

- Understands and obeys simple instructions, such as 'Don't touch', 'Come for dinner', 'Give me the ball'.

- Points to familiar persons, animals or toys when requested.

- Communicates wishes and needs by pointing and vocalising or screaming.

Social behaviour and play

- Pushes large, wheeled toy with handle on level ground.

- Explores properties and possibilities of toys, convenient household objects and sound-makers with lively interest.

- Engages in functional play, e.g., pushing toy car, pretends to drink from empty cup, bangs with toy hammer, etc.

- Carries dolls by limbs, hair or clothing. Repeatedly casts objects to floor in play or rejection and watches where things fall. Looks for hidden toy.

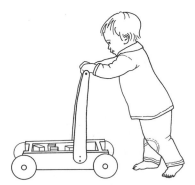

pushes large wheeled toy on level ground

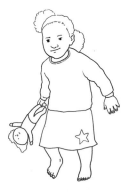

carries doll by leg

- Enjoys 'give and take' games, including initiating teasing by offering and then withdrawing an object. Physically restless and intensely curious regarding people, objects and events. Points to share interest.

- Emotionally labile and closely dependent upon adult's reassuring presence. Looks to care-giver to monitor his/her reactions, particularly in unfamiliar situations (social referencing) (Reddy et al. 1997). Is affectionate to familiar people.

Self care and independence

- Holds and drinks from a cup.

- Attempts to hold spoon, brings it to mouth and licks it but is unlikely to prevent it turning over.

- Chews well but continues to spill from mouth as lip closure not maintained.

- Helps more constructively with dressing.

- Needs constant supervision for protection against dangers owing to extended exploration of the environment.

AGE 18 MONTHS

Posture and large movements

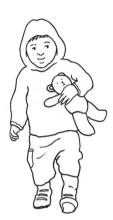

walks well carrying toy

■ Walks well with feet only slightly apart, starts and stops safely. No longer needs to hold upper arms in extension to balance. Runs rather stiffly though seldom falls.

■ Runs carefully, head held erect in midline, eyes fixed on ground 1–2 metres ahead but finds difficulty in negotiating obstacles.

■ Pushes and pulls large toys or boxes along the floor.

■ Can carry large doll or teddy bear while walking. Backs into small chair or slides in sideways to seat self.

■ Enjoys climbing and will climb forwards into adult's chair, then turn round and sit.

■ Walks upstairs with helping hand and sometimes downstairs. Creeps backwards downstairs or occasionally bumps down a few steps on buttocks facing forwards.

■ Kneels upright on flat surface without support. Flexes knees and hips in squatting position to pick up toy from floor and rises to feet using hands as support.

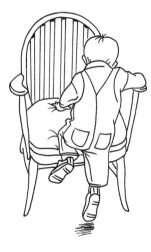

climbs into adult chair

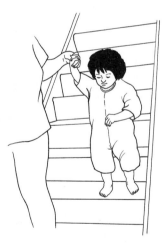

walks up and down stairs with help

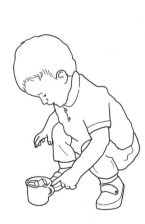

squats to pick up toy

- Picks up small objects immediately on sight with delicate pincer grasp. Recognises familiar people at a distance and points to distant interesting objects when outdoors.

- Enjoys simple picture books, often recognising and putting index finger on boldly coloured items on page. Turns several pages at a time.

- Holds pencil in mid- or upper shaft in whole hand in a pronated grip, or with crude approximation of thumb and fingers. Spontaneous to-and-fro scribble and dots, using either hand alone or sometimes with pencils in both hands.

- Builds tower of three cubes after demonstration and sometimes spontaneously. Enjoys putting small objects in and out of containers and learning the relative size of objects.

- Beginning to show preference for using one hand.

Visual perceptual and fine motor

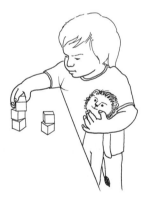 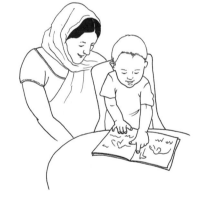

builds tower of three blocks *enjoys picture books*

- Chatters continually to self during play, with conversational intonation and emotional inflections.

- Listens and responds to spoken communications addressed directly to self. Uses between six and twenty recognisable words and understands many more. Echoes prominent or last word in short sentences addressed to self.

Speech, language and communication

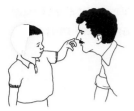

points to person's nose

- Demands a desired object by pointing accompanied by loud, urgent vocalisations or single words, checking back to adult that request has been noted.

- Enjoys nursery rhymes and tries to join in. Attempts to sing.

- Hands familiar objects to adult when requested (even if more than one option available). Obeys simple instructions, e.g., 'get your shoes' or 'shut the door'. Points to own, carer's or doll's hair, shoes, nose, feet.

Social behaviour and play

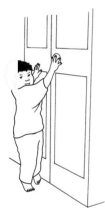

explores environment

- Explores environment energetically and with increasing understanding. No sense of danger.

- No longer takes toys to mouth.

- Treats dolls and teddies as babies, e.g., hugging, feeding, putting to bed, etc.

- Remembers where objects belong.

- Still casts objects to floor in play or anger, but less often and seldom troubles visually to verify arrival on target.

- Fascinated by household objects and imitates simple, everyday activities such as feeding doll, reading book, brushing floor, washing clothes.

- Plays contentedly alone but likes to be near familiar adult or older sibling. Emotionally still very dependent upon familiar adult, alternating between clinging and resistance.

- Exchanges toys, both cooperatively and in conflict, with peers.

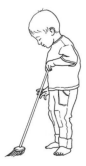

imitates everyday activities

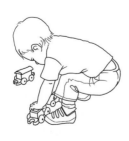

plays contendedly alone

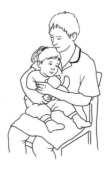

still dependent upon familiar adult

- Holds spoon and gets food safely to mouth, although may play with food. Holds cup between both hands and drinks without much spilling. Lifts cup alone but usually hands back to adult when finished.

- Assists with dressing and undressing, taking off shoes, socks and hat, but seldom able to replace.

- Beginning to give notice of urgent toilet needs by restlessness and vocalisation. Bowel control may be attained but very variable. May indicate wet or soiled pants.

Self-care and independence

AGE 2 YEARS

Posture and large movements

- Runs safely on whole foot, stopping and starting with ease and avoiding obstacles.

- Squats with complete steadiness to rest or to play with an object on the ground and rises to feet without using hands.

- Pushes and pulls large, wheeled toys easily forwards and usually able to walk backwards pulling handle. Pulls small wheeled toy by cord with obvious appreciation of direction.

- Climbs on furniture to look out of window or to open doors and can get down again.

- Shows increasing understanding of size of self in relation to size and position of objects in the environment and to enclosed spaces such as a cupboard or cardboard box.

- Walks upstairs and downstairs holding on to rail or wall, two feet to a step.

- Throws small ball overhand and forwards, without falling over. Walks into large ball when trying to kick it.

- Sits on small tricycle but cannot use pedals. Propels vehicle forwards with feet on floor.

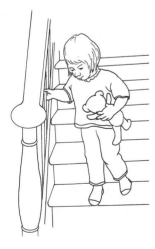

walks up and down stairs

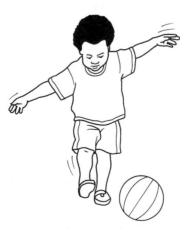

walks into large ball

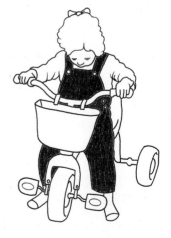

sits and steers tricycle, cannot yet use pedals

■ Good manipulative skills; picks up tiny objects accurately and quickly and places down neatly with increasing skill. Can match square, circular and triangular shapes in a simple jigsaw.

■ Holds a pencil well down shaft towards point, using thumb and first two fingers. Mostly uses preferred hand.

■ Spontaneous circular scribble as well as to-and-fro scribble and dots; imitates vertical line and sometimes 'V' shape.

■ Builds tower of six or seven cubes.

■ Enjoys picture books, recognising fine details in favourite pictures. Turns pages singly. Can name and match pictures with toys or with other pictures.

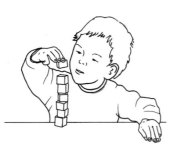
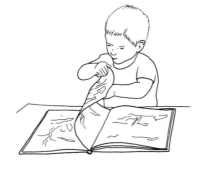
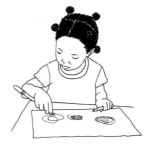

builds tower of six or seven blocks   *enjoys books, turns pages singly*   *holds pencil and scribbles*

■ Recognises familiar adults in photograph after once shown, but not usually self as yet.

■ Binocular vision at this age can be tested with Kay Pictures Vision Test.

Speech, language and communication

■ Uses fifty or more recognisable words appropriately and understands many more. Puts two or more words together to form simple sentences.

■ Attends to communications addressed to self and begins to listen with obvious interest to more general conversation. Refers to self by name and talks to self continually in long monologues during play but may be incomprehensible to others.

- Echolalia almost constant, with one or more stressed words repeated.

- Constantly asking names of objects and people.

- Joins in nursery rhymes and action songs.

- Indicates hair, hand, feet, nose, eyes, mouth, shoes, etc., in pictures. Names familiar objects and pictures.

- Carries out simple instructions such as 'Go and see what the postman has brought'. Follows a series of two simple but related commands, e.g., 'Get your teddy and put it in the bag'.

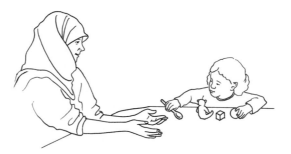

hands familiar objects to adults on request

Social behaviour and play

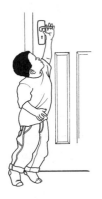

turns door handle, has little comprehension of dangers

- Follows parent or carer around house and imitates domestic activities in simultaneous play. Intensely curious regarding environment. Turns door handles and often runs outside. Little comprehension of common dangers.

- Spontaneously engages in simple role or situational make-believe activities. Beginning to show meaningful short play sequence and definition-by-use of doll's-house-sized toys. Substitutes one item for another, e.g., pretends a brick is a car.

- Constantly demanding parent's or carer's attention. Clings tightly in affection, fatigue or fear, although resistive and rebellious when thwarted. Tantrums when frustrated or in trying to make self understood, but attention is usually readily distracted.

- Defends own possessions with determination.

- May take turns but, as yet, has little idea of sharing either toys or the attention of adults.

- Parallel play present; plays contentedly near other children but not with them.

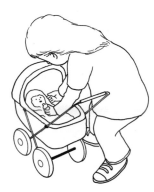

engages in make-believe play

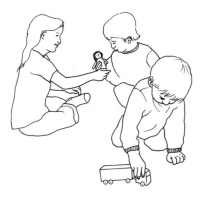

plays near others but not with them

- Resentful of attention shown to other children, particularly by own familiars.

- Unwilling to defer or modify immediate satisfaction of wishes.

- Feeds self competently with a spoon but is easily distracted. Controlled biting on biscuits. Chews with lips closed, some spillage. Lifts cup and drinks well without spilling and replaces cup on table without difficulty. Asks for food and drink.

- Puts on hat and shoes.

- Usually attempts to verbalise toilet needs in reasonable time, but still unreliable.

Self-care skills and independence

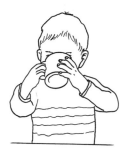

lifts cup and drinks well without spillage

AGE 2½ YEARS

Posture and large movements

■ Runs well and climbs easy nursery apparatus. Walks upstairs confidently and downstairs holding rail, two feet to a step.

■ Pushes and pulls large toys skilfully but may have difficulty in steering them around obstacles.

■ Can jump with two feet together from a low step. Can stand on tiptoe if shown.

■ Throws ball from hand somewhat stiffly at body level. Kicks large ball but gently and lopsidedly.

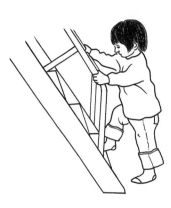

climbs play equipment

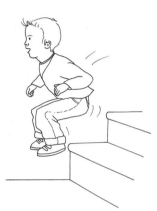

jumps from bottom step, both feet together

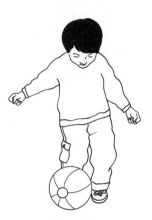

kicks large ball gently

Visual perception and fine motor

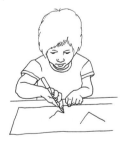

holds pencil in preferred hand and imitates 'v'

■ Recognises minute details in picture books. Recognises self in photographs once shown.

■ Builds tower of seven-plus cubes using preferred hand. Inserts square, circular and triangular shapes in a jigsaw by recognising the shape. Begins to correct the orientation of the shapes from 33 months.

■ Holds pencil in preferred hand, with improved tripod grasp. Imitates horizontal line and circle, and usually 'T' and 'V'.

- Uses 200 or more recognisable words, but speech shows numerous immaturities of articulation and sentence structure.

- Usually intelligible to familiar carers.

- Knows full name.

- Talks audibly and intelligibly to self at play, concerning events happening here and now.

- Continues to imitate phrases (echolalia).

- Can select pictures of actions, e.g., 'Which one shows eating?'.

- Recognises general family name categories, e.g., 'baby', 'mother', 'granny', etc.

- Makes frequent comments on objects and events of interest, directed to care-givers.

- Continually asking questions beginning 'What?' or 'Who?'. Uses pronouns 'I', 'me' and 'you' correctly.

- Stuttering in eagerness common. Says a few nursery rhymes. Enjoys simple familiar stories read from picture book.

- Plays meaningfully with miniature doll's house-size toys, adding an intelligent, running commentary.

- Requires physical or verbal prompts in order to switch attention to looking and listening if engrossed in play.

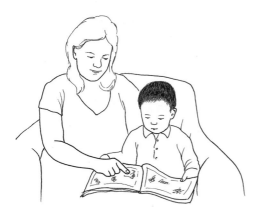

enjoys simple familiar stories in picture books

Social behaviour and play

- Exceedingly active, restless and resistive of restraint. Has little understanding of common dangers or need to defer immediate wishes.

- Throws tantrums when thwarted and is less easily distracted.

- Emotionally still very dependent on adult and requires reassurance in unfamiliar situations.

- More sustained role play, such as putting dolls to bed, washing clothes, driving cars, but with frequent reference to a friendly adult.

- Acts out common activities using substituted materials, e.g., has pretend tea parties, with gravel on plates to represent food.

- Watches other children at play with interest, occasionally joining in for a few minutes but, as yet, has little notion of the necessity to share playthings or adults' attention.

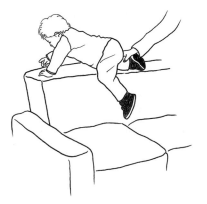

active and curious with little notion of common dangers

Self-care and independence

- Eats skilfully with spoon and may use a fork.

- Pulls down pants when using the toilet but seldom is able to replace them.

- May be dry through the night, although this is extremely variable.

- Walks alone up stairs using alternating feet one foot to each step, comes down stairs two feet to a step and can carry large toy. Usually jumps from bottom step with two feet together.

- Climbs nursery apparatus with agility.

- Can turn around obstacles and corners while running and also while pushing and pulling large toys. Walks forwards, backwards, sideways, etc., hauling large toys with complete confidence.

- Obviously appreciates size and movements of own body in relation to external objects and space.

- Rides tricycle using pedals and can steer it round wide corners.

walks up and down stairs, carrying large toy

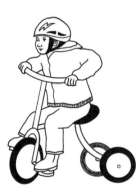

rides tricycle, using pedals

- Can stand and walk on tiptoe. Can stand momentarily on one (preferred) foot when shown.

- Can sit with feet crossed at ankles.

- Can throw a ball overhand and catch large ball on or between extended arms. Kicks ball forcibly.

- Builds tower of nine or ten cubes; by 3½ years builds one or more bridges of three cubes from a model using two hands cooperatively. Threads large wooden beads on shoelace.

- Can close fist and wiggle thumb in imitation, right and left. Holds pencil near the point in preferred hand, between the first two fingers and thumb, and uses it with good control. Copies circle,

Visual perceptual and fine motor

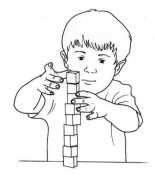

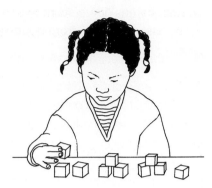

builds tower of nine or ten blocks

builds three-block bridges from a model

also letters 'V', 'H' and 'T'. Imitates a cross. Draws person with head and usually adds one or two other features or parts.

■ Matches two or three primary colours, usually red and yellow, but may confuse blue and green. May know names of colours.

■ Enjoys painting with large brush on easel, covering whole paper with wash of colour or painting primitive 'pictures', which are usually named during or after production.

■ Cuts with toy scissors.

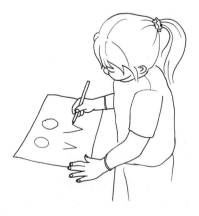

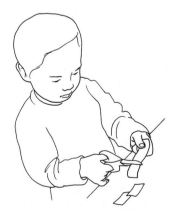

copies circle and letter 'v'

cuts with scissors

- Speech modulating in loudness and range of pitch. Large vocabulary intelligible even to strangers, but speech still contains many immature sound substitutions and unconventional grammatical forms.

- Gives full name and sex and, sometimes, age. Uses personal pronouns and plurals correctly and also most prepositions.

- Still talks to self in long monologues, mostly concerned with the immediate present, particularly during make-believe activities. Carries on simple conversations and able to describe briefly present activities and past experiences.

- Asks many questions beginning 'What?', 'Where? and 'Who?'.

- Can identify objects by function, e.g., 'Which one do we eat with?'. Understands descriptive concepts such as 'big', 'wet', 'hot', 'the same', etc.

- Listens eagerly to stories and demands favourites over and over again. Knows several nursery rhymes to repeat and sometimes sing.

- Counts by rote up to ten or more, but little appreciation of quantity beyond two or three.

Speech, language and communication

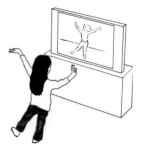

enjoys watching television, will join in action songs

- General behaviour is more amenable – can be affectionate and confiding.

- Vividly realised make-believe play, including invented people and objects.

- Enjoys playing on the floor with bricks, boxes, toy trains and dolls, etc., alone or in company with siblings.

- Joins in active make-believe play with other children. Understands sharing playthings.

- Shows affection for younger siblings.

- Shows some appreciation of difference between present and past and of the need to defer satisfaction of wishes to the future.

Social behaviour and play

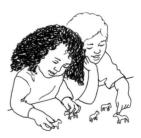

joins in make-believe play with other children

Self-care and independence

- Eats with a fork and spoon.

- Washes hands but needs adult supervision with drying. Can pull pants down and up but needs help with buttons and other fastenings.

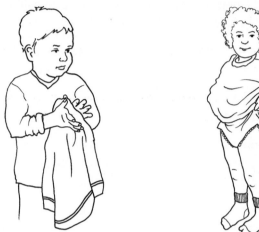

washes hands but needs supervision with drying

can pull pants down and up

- May be dry through the night, although this is very variable.

- Likes to help adults with domestic activities including gardening, shopping, etc.

- Makes an effort to keep surroundings tidy.

- Walks or runs alone up and down stairs, one foot to a step in adult fashion. Navigates self-locomotion skilfully, turning sharp corners, running, pushing and pulling.

- Climbs ladders and trees.

- Can stand, walk and run on tiptoe.

- Expert rider of tricycle, executing sharp U-turns easily.

- Stands on one (preferred) foot for 3–5 seconds and hops on preferred foot.

- Arranges and picks up objects from floor by bending from waist with knees extended.

- Sits with knees crossed.

- Shows increasing skill in ball games, throwing, catching, bouncing, kicking, etc., including use of bat.

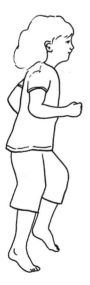

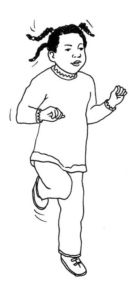

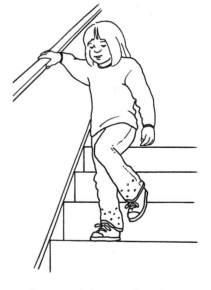

can stand or run on tiptoe *hops on one foot* *walks up and down stairs, one foot to a step*

Visual perceptual and fine motor

■ Builds tower of ten or more cubes and several bridges of three from one model on request or spontaneously. Builds three steps with six cubes after demonstration.

■ Imitates spreading of hand and bringing thumb into opposition with each finger in turn, right and left.

■ Holds and uses pencil in a dynamic tripod grasp with good control, like adults. Copies cross and also letters 'V', 'H', 'T' and 'O'. Draws a person with head, legs and trunk and, usually, arms and fingers. Draws a recognisable house on request or spontaneously.

■ Beginning to name drawings before production.

■ Matches and names four primary colours correctly.

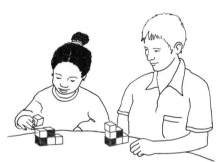

builds three steps after demonstration

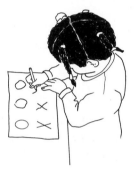

copies circles and crosses

Speech, language and communication

■ Speech grammatically correct and completely intelligible. Shows only a few immature sound substitutions, usually of r-l-w-y group, p-th-f-s group or k-t sound group. May simplify consonant clusters, e.g., 'sring' for 'string'. Gives connected account of recent events and experiences. Gives full name, home address and usually age.

■ Eternally asking questions 'Why?', 'When?', 'How?', and meanings of words.

- Understands some abstract concepts, e.g., 'one of', 'before' and 'after', 'if'.

- Listens to and tells long stories, sometimes confusing fact and fantasy.

- Counts by rote up to twenty or more, and beginning to count objects by word and touch in one-to-one correspondence up to four or five.

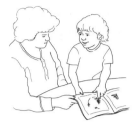

enjoys listening to and telling stories

- Enjoys jokes and verbal incongruities.

- Knows several nursery rhymes and can repeat or sing correctly.

- General behaviour more independent and strongly self-willed.

- Inclined to verbal impertinence with adults and quarrelling with playmates when wishes crossed.

- Shows sense of humour in talk and social activities.

- Dramatic make-believe play and dressing-up favoured. Floor games very complicated but habits less tidy.

- Constructive out-of-doors building with any materials available.

- Needs companionship of other children with whom he/she is alternately cooperative and aggressive, as with adults, but understands need to argue with words rather than blows. Understands taking turns as well as sharing.

- Shows concern for younger siblings and sympathy for play-mates in distress.

- Appreciates past, present and future time.

Social behaviour and play

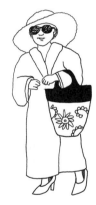

imaginative dressing-up play

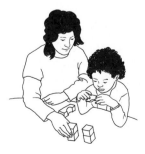

understands need for taking turns in play

Self-care and independence

■ Eats skilfully with spoon and fork. Spreads butter on bread with a knife.

■ Washes and dries hands. Brushes teeth. Can undress and dress except for laces, ties and back buttons.

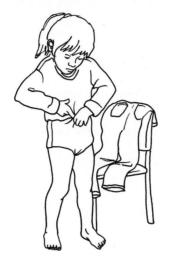

*dresses and
undresses alone*

- Walks easily on narrow line. Runs lightly on toes. Active and skilful in climbing, sliding, swinging, digging and doing various 'stunts'. Skips on alternate feet.

- Can stand on one foot for 8–10 seconds, right or left, and usually also stands on preferred foot, with arms folded. Can hop 2 or 3 metres forwards on each foot separately.

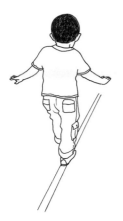

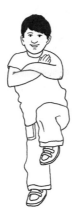

walks on narrow line　　*stands on one foot, arms folded*

- Moves rhythmically to music.

- Grips strongly with either hand.

- Can bend and touch toes without flexing knees.

- Throws and catches a ball well, though catching with one hand does not develop until 9–10 years. Plays all varieties of ball games with considerable ability, including those requiring appropriate placement or scoring, according to accepted rules.

- Picks up and replaces minute objects.

- Builds elaborate models when shown, such as three steps with six cubes from model; sometimes four steps from ten cubes. Holds the cubes with the ulnar fingers tucked in and the hand diagonal to get a better view.

Visual perceptual and fine motor

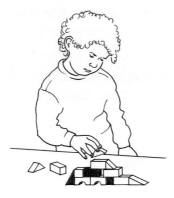

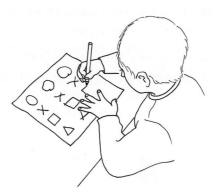

constructs elaborate models   *copies squares and triangles*

■ Good control in writing and drawing with pencils and paint brushes. Copies square and, at 5½ years, a triangle. Also copies letters 'V' , 'T' , 'H', 'O', 'X', 'L', 'A', 'C', 'U' and 'Y'. Writes a few letters spontaneously.

■ Draws recognisable man with head, trunk, legs, arms and features. Draws house with door, windows, roof and chimney.

■ Can cut a strip of paper neatly.

■ Spontaneously produces many other pictures containing several items and usually indication of background of environment, and names before production.

■ Colours pictures neatly, staying within outlines.

■ Counts fingers on one hand with index finger of other.

■ Names four or more primary colours and matches ten or twelve colours.

Speech, language and communication

■ Speech fluent, grammatically conventional and usually phonetically correct except for confusions of s-f-th group.

■ Loves to be read or told stories and acts them out in detail later, alone or with friends.

■ Gives full name, age and usually birthday. Gives home address.

■ Defines concrete nouns by use.

- Understands time and sequence concepts and uses terms such as 'first', 'then', 'last'.

- Constantly asks meaning of abstract words and uses them, usually appropriately but with some errors.

- Delights in reciting or singing rhymes and jingles. Enjoys jokes and riddles.

Social behaviour and play

- Developing self-regulation. General behaviour more sensible, controlled and independent with wide variability in different situations.

- Follows tidiness routines but needs constant reminders.

- Domestic and dramatic play continued alone or with playmates from day to day.

- Plays imaginatively, creating scenes using miniatures. Substitutes unrelated objects in play, e.g., pretends a brick is an apple.

- Plans and builds constructively in and out of doors.

- Chooses own friends. Can play cooperatively with peers most of the time and understands need for rules and fair play.

- Shows definite sense of humour.

- Appreciates meaning of time in relation to daily programme.

- Tender and protective towards younger children and pets. Comforts playmates in distress.

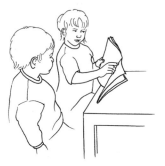

affectionate and helpful to younger children

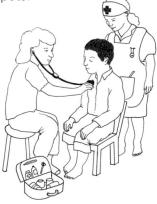

dramatic play with peers

Self-care and independence

- Uses knife and fork competently.

- Washes and dries face and hands but needs help or supervision for the rest. Undresses and dresses alone.

Assessing Children's Developmental Progress

General Principles of Assessment

Child development is a dynamic process through which a child is transformed from reacting to sensations and being dependent on carers to making sense of information and responding in a planned, organised and independent manner. This process does not simply unfold with neurological maturation but is shaped, positively or negatively, by the interactions between biological and environmental influences (Figure 1). These interactions result in a high level of variability in children's developmental outcomes. Learning about both the sequences of development and the context of development, is necessary for understanding developmental problems and for planning interventions.

Understanding the process of child development

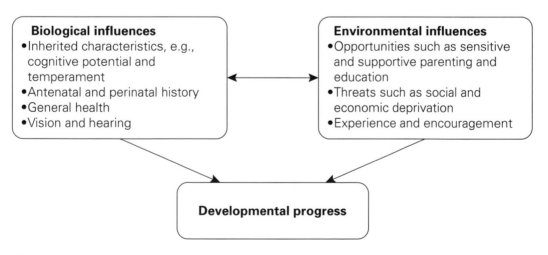

Figure 1 *Influences on development.*

Milestones, variations and disorders of development

Children's developmental milestones are convenient guidelines to look at the rate or the extent of their progress. Even though the sequences of developmental milestones are similar in most children, there is a wide individual variation in the rate of achievement, largely attributable to the factors outlined in Figure 1. Developmental disorders generally present with:

- qualitative abnormality: poor awareness of task and context, slowness in completing a task, poor social interest or presence of associated behaviours and movements;

- disordered developmental sequence: e.g., infant who is easier to stand than sit, language expression better than understanding, hyperlexia (advanced reading) coexisting with poor language;

- severely delayed rate of development: e.g., not sitting by 10 months, not walking by 18 months or no single words by 18 months;

- regression of development: losing previously acquired skill.

Developmental examination

History taking

Parental concerns are best elicited using a combination of open-ended questions and asking for examples of behaviour in each domain of development. Parents are good at observing and reporting current behaviours, if the right questions are asked, though their interpretation of why their child does something may be incorrect. Information regarding family history, family and social environment and the pre-, peri- and post-natal history should be obtained. Children's current general health and a history of illness or medication may be relevant to their current presentation.

Observation and assessment

Observations made during free-play situations are a rich source of information about children's developmental progress. A suitable selection of toys and an interactive style is essential. Toys should be both age appropriate and relevant to the developmental domains, for example:

- cause-and-effect relation (pop-up toys), means-end relation (a toy on wheel attached to a string), exploration and imitation behaviour (bell);

- functional play (cup/spoon, doll/brush) and pretend play (doll/teddy/tea set)

- fine motor/eye–hand coordination (bricks, crayons, pencil/paper, shape sorter and puzzles – form boards);

- language and play (books at different levels, large and miniature toys).

During the assessment, a combination of supportive interaction with the child and time for the child to play or solve a problem on his/her own gives information about the child's awareness, interests, attention, ability to organise self, initiate interaction and respond to the examiner's approaches, in addition to gross and fine motor skills. It is crucial to look at not only *what* the child does but *how* the child does it – the quality of function in response to an individual task demand should be observed. A range of structured assessments are available for gathering normative developmental information in a standardised manner, which is sometimes required for diagnostic or monitoring purposes.

Making sense of a child's developmental progress requires observing the child's achievements against the developmental norms, consideration of the qualitative aspects of the child's functioning, and other child- and context-related factors. Developmental charts (Section 1) can provide mean age equivalents for achieved milestones. Informal assessments of development are often erroneous, and full information from history, observation/assessment and physical examination (Box 1) must be considered for making a diagnostic interpretation. As a general rule, developmental delay is described as moderate where the developmental age is between two-thirds and half and severe when it is less then half of the chronological age. However, it may be more informative to describe a child's strengths and difficulties to highlight needs, rather than using the terms 'severe' or 'moderate', as these are open to misinterpretation.

Developmental diagnosis

Development is a dynamic process, and each child is continually striving for adaptation within the given biological and environmental

> **BOX 1** Physical examination
>
> ■ Dysmorphic features and congenital malformation that may suggest a particular syndrome or aetiology such as foetal alcohol syndrome.
>
> ■ Examination of skin for pigmented and hypopigmented marks (e.g., neurofibromatosis or tuberous sclerosis).
>
> ■ Growth: measure head circumference, height and weight.
>
> ■ Vision and hearing: observe visual and hearing behaviour. Arrange orthoptic and or ophthalmologic assessment/audiological assessment.
>
> ■ Neurological examination: tone, movements, reflexes, power and any abnormal movements. Observe for any asymmetry of findings.

constraints (Sroufe 1983). Repeated observations in different settings may be required for interpretation. A narrow focus on the child's abilities in one particular domain, without attention to situational effects and task demands, abilities in other domains and to the family and social context, is likely to lead to a wrong conclusion such as diagnosing developmental delay in the presence of sensory impairment or poor social adaptation.

Further reading

Bee, H. and Boyd D. (2007) *The Developing Child*. Boston, Mass.: Pearson.
Siegler, R., Deloache, J., Eisenberg, N. (2003) *How Children Develop*. New York: Worth.

Motor development

The progress in motor development is the result of an ongoing bi-directional interaction between maturation and experience dependent factors, which results in a continually self-organising dynamic system (Thelen 1995) (see Figure 2).

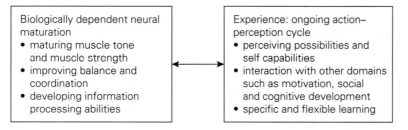

Figure 2 *Influences on motor development.*

Children's motor developmental progress can be viewed in five phases, with experience playing an increasingly significant role through this progress (Galluhe and Ozmum 2006) (see Table 1).

Identification of disorders of motor development requires moving away from an over-reliance on the milestones of development, which have a wide range of variability, to a framework that includes:

Identification of potential disorders of motor development

1. qualitative observations of:

    (a) static (at rest) and dynamic (on movement) posture and balance;
    (b) associated movements;

2. common variations in achieving locomotor abilities;
3. neurological and other markers of abnormalities.

Table 1 Phases of motor development.

Birth–4 months	■ Primitive reflexive movements.	
4 months–1 year	■ Inhibition of primitive reflexes by 6 months. ■ Improving muscle tone with reducing flexor muscle tone in the limbs and improving extensor tone in the trunk. ■ Improving postural control and balance. ■ Movements become differentiated and functional such as reaching, grasping, sitting, walking.	Primarily maturation-dependent progress
1–2 years	■ Better differentiated and more precise movements. ■ Improving stability and power.	
2–7 years	■ Maturing functional movements such as running, jumping, catching, throwing, writing, cutting. ■ Improving rhythm, sequence, integration and flow to achieve efficient, co-ordinated and controlled performance in day to day activities.	Increasing significance of experience
7 years onwards	■ Applying motor skills to specialised activities of sports and work.	

Static Posture and balance

Observe the infant in supine, pull to sit, supported sitting, prone and supported standing (see Table 2) for posture, balance and range of movements.

Table 2 Static posture and balance development.

			Mean ages (months)
Head control	Supine	Turns head sideways to track objects	1
	Supine	Lifts head up	5
	Pull to sit	Slight head lag	4
	Sitting	Holds head steady	3 (3–4)
	Prone	Lifts head up fully (30–45 degrees)	3
Trunk posture	Sitting	Balanced with straight spine	7 (5–9)
Limbs: range of movements	Arms	Full extension	2
	Legs	Popletial angle: 90/110/150 degrees	2/5/9
Hand posture	Supine	Hands mostly open	2 (1–3)

Based on: Frankenburgh et al. (1975), Piek (2006), Amiel-Tison and Grenier (1986).

Observations of dynamic posture include base of support and balance and arm and leg posture while standing, walking or running.

The base of support decreases with age, and legs are in line with the body while standing by the age of 4 years. The balance similarly improves, enabling children to walk on a straight line by 3 years and stand on one foot briefly by 5 years.

When infants start walking, they hold their arms spread out in a rather rigid manner. By age 2 years, most children move their arms reciprocally, and by the age of 4 years the arms are by the child's side and move reciprocally. Infants hold their legs apart, slightly flexed at knees, feet turned outwards and make a flat-footed contact with the ground on walking. By the age of 18 months, they achieve a heel-toe contact with the ground, the base narrows, and the outward rotation is minimal.

Healthy infants spend about 5 per cent of their waking time making repetitive movements, such as swaying of body, waving of arms, kicking the legs, banging of objects or bouncing up and down, which may have a promoting role for neuro-muscular coordination. Most of these movements reach a peak between 4 and 7 months and decline by the end of the first year. Persistence of these movements beyond 18 months of age and presence of excessive repetitive movements at any age may be an indicator of neuro-developmental abnormalities.

Children's muscle tone, their preferred resting posture in infancy (prefers to lie on tummy or back) and their family history may have a significant impact on developmental sequence and the age of achieving independent walking (Table 3).

Dynamic posture and balance

Base of support and balance

Arm and leg posture on walking

Repetitive movements

Common variations in achieving locomotor abilities

Table 3 Common variations in achieving locomotion.

	Sit Mean/97% (months)	Crawl Mean/97% (months)	Walk Mean/97% (months)
Crawling (Normal tone) 83%	7/9	9/13	13/18
Stand and walk (Prefer to lie on back) 6%	7/11		11/14
Bottom shuffling (Low muscle tone) 9%	12/15		17/28
Creeping/rolling (Low muscle tone) 1%	9/12	12/17	18/27

Adapted from Robson (1984).

Neurological and other markers that indicate abnormality

Eliciting developmentally appropriate symptoms and signs (Table 4) helps identify infants requiring further detailed assessment.

Table 4 Markers that indicate abnormality.

First 4 months	5–8 months	9–12 months	13 months–5 years
■ Irritability. ■ Feeding/respiratory problems. ■ Floppiness or stiffness. ■ Poor head control.	■ Asymmetry of movements. ■ Persisting primitive reflexes; fisted hands. ■ Hypotonia. ■ Poor eye movements.	■ Poor trunk control. ■ Poor supporting reflexes. ■ Poor balance. ■ Not sitting by 10 months. ■ Poor hand function. ■ Hypo/hypertonia.	■ Poor balance. ■ Stiffness on movements (dynamic hypertonia) toe walking or legs crossing. ■ Poor co-ordination. ■ Not walking by 18 months.

Other findings such as unusual movements, weakness, fluctuating tone, rigidness of movement, large or small head, spinal abnormality, history of epilepsy, may also indicate abnormality at any age.

Having a good scheme for making observations, a schedule of development for referencing the findings, a detailed history of the child to include feeding and respiratory problems, family and the environment and a complete neuro-motor examination, is often required to identify possible abnormality, in the context of a wide range of variation in the developmental norms, without raising undue anxiety or giving false reassurance.

Making sense of findings

All aspects of children's development benefit from opportunities and encouragement to explore. Most children do not need any special considerations for their motor development. Children with a vulnerability of neurological maturation benefit from enhanced opportunities, instructions and encouragement, and suitable guidance from a physiotherapist should be obtained. Developmentally appropriate, organised physical activities help children improve in their skills and their general strength, agility and motivation.

Supporting motor development

Amiel-Tison, A. and Grenier, A (1986) *Neurological Assessment during the First Year of Life*. Oxford: Oxford University Press.
Galluhe, D. I. and Ozmum, J. C. (2006) *Understanding Motor Development*. London: McGraw-Hill.
Piek, J. P. (2006) *Infant Motor Development*. Champaign, Ill.: Human Kinetics.

Further reading

Visual-perceptual and fine motor development

Children change from reacting to sensations and making random and uncoordinated movements to acting in a planned and coordinated manner. This enables them to reach, pick up and play with toys, catch, throw and kick balls and manage day-to-day activities of using spoon and fork, dressing and undressing themselves, and learning to write (see Figure 3).

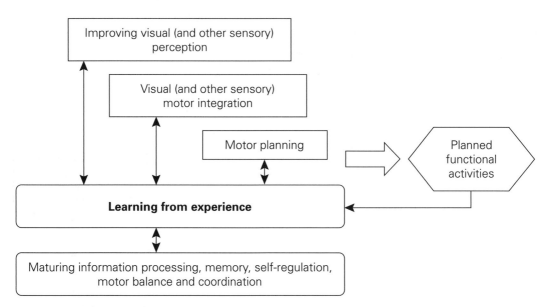

Figure 3 *Influences on fine motor development.*

From sensation to perception

Children gain information about the world through various sensations: vision, hearing, touch, taste, smell and sensation of movement (kinaesthetic). Sensations become perception when they are connected with stored information and take on meaning to guide thinking and action. Any action generates more information which further guides thinking and action forming an action–perception loop (Figure 3).

Development of visual perception is apparent in social functioning (Figure 4) and in the infant's emerging ability to search and find, reach out and grasp and manipulate objects (Figure 5).

Visual perception

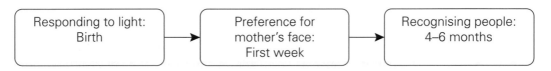

Figure 4 *Progression of visual recognition.*

Infants begin to make sense of object unity (that visible parts of objects are connected) from 3 months and look for partially hidden objects by 6 months. However, it is not until about 9 months that they begin to retrieve completely covered objects. By about 12 months they can track an object's hidden movement, so that when

Finding objects

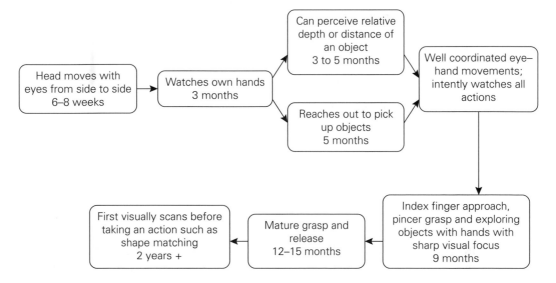

Figure 5 *Combining visual perception with fine motor development: reaching, grasping and manipulating.*

a moving toy goes under a table, they anticipate that it will come out at the other end.

Improving perceptual-motor coordination

Gradual improvement in finger perceptual discrimination is apparent in improving ability to do the finger-to-finger or thumb–finger opposition tasks up to about the age of 4 years in most children, and by the age of 5 years, nearly all children can do this task if demonstrated. By now, they are able to make movements that cross the body midline with ease. From the fourth year onward, children begin to integrate their perceptual, motor and verbal abilities. They are able to have a conversation while doing different activities such as using knives and forks. They gradually become interested in using the fine motor skills for art and craft activities with increasing sophistication.

> **BOX 2** Handedness
>
> Some lateral bias in head position or hand preference is apparent early during infancy. Stable handedness appears gradually from 2 to 4 years and is apparent in tasks involving the use of crayon and construction activities with bricks. Early appearance of 'fixed' or strong handedness or ignoring the use of the other hand may indicate neurological abnormality.
>
> Around 10 per cent of people are left-handed. Like any other group of children, left-handed children have wide variation in their learning and other abilities. However, left-handed children have to make more adjustments in day-to-day life as almost everything is designed for use by right-handed people and this may be reflected in some functional areas such as writing. It is wrong to attribute a child's difficulties to handedness without careful evaluation.

Motor-planning refers to an ability to chain together a series of actions into a purposeful action in an efficient way. Children may well understand what is required from a task and have the muscle strength and movements (i.e., they do not have any known neurological impairment of movement or posture) to do the individual components of the task and yet be unable, or find it difficult, to carry out the full sequence. Simple daily tasks such as tying shoelaces can be confusing if the planning ability is weak. Such problems with motor planning may indicate developmental coordination disorder or dyspraxia.

From random to planned movements

Children find it easier to copy an action after demonstration, and making an individual movement is easier than a series of movements. With age, motor planning is helped by improving attention to demonstrations, improving ability to look at the part and the whole and the positive feedback they get every time a targeted action is achieved. Memory helps the development of motor skills as more successful patterns of activities are retained and applied.

Children's drawings reflect their fine motor skills, perceptual awareness of the world around them and their representational skills. Initial drawing skills progress from making random marks on paper by 12–15 months, a vigorous to-and-fro scribble by 15–18 months to making circular scribble by the age of 24 months. By 30 months, more intentional circular scribble or immature circles emerge. Toddlers often vocalise while scribbling, as if they were giving a running commentary. The act of drawing and the running commentary together seems to have a meaning. By the age of 4, more angles are seen in children's drawings, and they are able to copy a cross and, by 4½ years, a square. At the age of 5 years, children make a clear and accurate cross, the lines become straighter, and angles become sharper. The ability to copy geometric forms, particularly the oblique cross, is seen as an indication of writing readiness in the young child, as it requires crossing the body midline. Towards the end of the fifth year, children are beginning to make three-dimensional representations in their drawings, such as drawing the base of a cylinder.

Children's drawings

Drawing human figures

At around 3–4 years of age, children begin to draw pictures with recognisable features – the most common subject being a human figure. In general, children begin with drawing circles with marks in or around them, proceed to draw arms and then legs projecting directly from the circle by 3 years, then add another circle as a body and more parts at about 4½ years, and the limbs are drawn in two dimensions or width by the age of 5½–6 years.

> **BOX 3** Handwriting
>
> At about 4 years of age, when children copy letters these are often scattered on the page with no stable baseline and are often placed on their sides and maybe slanted to varying degrees. Letters with horizontal and vertical strokes (H, I, T) are easier for the young child to replicate than letters with slanted lines, or those combining curved and slanted lines (D, Z, G, N). Many 5-year-old children are able to print their first name and by the age of 6 most children can print the alphabet, their first and last names. About 50–60 per cent of children from the age of 5–6 years may reverse numbers and letters in a variety of ways and only about 10 per cent are still doing this by the age of 7. The quality of handwriting develops quickly during 6–9 years, in that handwriting becomes automatic, organised, and is available to facilitate the development of ideas.

Associated movements

Two- to 3-year-old children normally curl their hands up while running or trying to walk on their heels or toes and move their tongue in and out while drawing or cutting. Most of these associated movements gradually disappear by the age of 7 years, though increasing the difficulty or the stress of the task makes some associated movements appear even in adults. Persistence of these movements or when these movements in some way create difficulty in carrying out age expected functional tasks would require further assessment.

Children with fine motor difficulties are slow to acquire most day-to-day activities of self-care such as dressing/undressing, buttoning, tying shoelaces or managing a spoon or fork and are often described as bumping into things, knocking things over and not being able to 'keep up' with others in playground activities. At school, they have delayed and poor writing skills and a poor ability to plan activities that others find relatively easy. Many children with poor fine-motor activities also have poor attention to task and are overactive. Such difficulties often lead to poor self-esteem and poor social skills and behaviour difficulties, further increasing their isolation from their peer group.

Parents and teachers are often the first to pick up cues of possible fine-motor difficulties. A good starting point is having a range of questions to gather information from parents and teachers regarding the broad aspects of functional difficulties as described above. Such information is valuable in identifying children who would benefit from further assessment and advice from an occupational therapist.

Presentation of fine-motor difficulties

Parents and teachers can help the child by acknowledging the child's difficulty and by applying some general methods to improve the child's functional performance.

Supporting fine-motor development

■ Give simple step-by-step instructions for the task.

■ Demonstrate or model activities.

■ Model the activity by verbalising steps aloud.

■ Allow time for practice.

■ Set up a variety of activities.

■ Use pictures or written lists to organise activities.

■ Reorganise and label things to make them easy for the child to find.

■ Consider changing physical environment such as using Velcro, thicker pencils, stable paper pads and adjusting the height of chair/desk.

Further reading

Cermak, S. A. and Larkin D. (2002) *Developmental Coordination Disorder*. Albany, NY: Delmar Thomson Learning.

Cratty, J. B. (1986) *Perceptual and Motor Development in Infants and Children*, 3rd edn. Englewood Cliffs, NJ: Prentice Hall.

Communication

Typically developing children are highly competent communicators well before the appearance of recognisable words. By the end of the first year, children can attract and direct an adult's attention, indicate a range of emotions, make clear requests and even make comments or ask questions using a range of non-verbal communication strategies.

Language is a cognitive process that develops in a social context; i.e., it is acquired through interaction with caring and responsive adults rather than through formal instruction. Learning and use of language are influenced by the interaction of biological, cognitive, psycho-social and environmental factors (Figure 6).

How is communication learned?

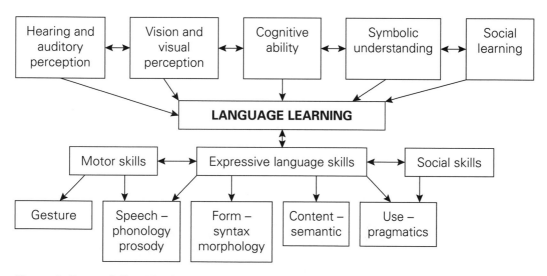

Figure 6 *Factors influencing language learning.*

Table 5 Aspects of speech, language and communication.

Speech	Production of sounds
Phonology	The system of consonants and vowels that make up a language
Syntax/grammar	The way that words and parts of words combine in phrases and sentences
Morphology	The changes made at word level to convey specific meanings
Semantics	The meaning of sentences, words and parts of words
Pragmatics	How language is used in social situations
Prosody	The rhythm (stress) and music (intonation) of speech
Receptive skills	Understanding of language
Expressive skills	Using speech and language to communicate

As with other aspects of development, there is considerable variation in the age at which children reach specific milestones, but most show similarities in the overall sequence, even across languages. There may be differences in rates of acquisition and in learning styles, and dissociations between components may occur; e.g., some children may be slow to master the sound system of the language whilst achieving typical grammatical milestones.

BOX 4 Joint Attention

The development of joint attention is a key stage in learning to communicate. The attentional focus of the young infant is the faces of responsive adults and older children. At around 5 months external objects and events become main interest before, at around 9 months, interactions include another person to become triadic (infant-object-other) (Bruner 1983). Index-finger pointing becomes established just before the first birthday. The ability to follow an adult's eyes/finger pointing, and to direct another's attention to things of interest allows a child to learn the connections between language heard and the objects/events/concepts it represents (mapping).

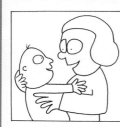 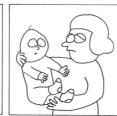 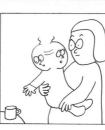 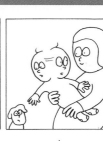

attention to
people

attention to
things

requesting

commenting

Failure to develop joint attention and pretend play behaviours by 18 months has been shown to be highly correlated with childhood autism. Whilst not diagnostic, delayed skills in this area may indicate the need for further neuro-developmental assessment (Baird et al. 2000).

Assessing speech, language and communication

The majority of parents can provide accurate description of their child's current level of functioning given appropriate prompts. Questions such as 'How much does your child understand?' tend to produce the unhelpful response 'Everything', because parents are highly skilled in unknowingly scaffolding interactions so the child is successful. Children also make sense of the situational non-verbal cues their carers provide when addressing young children (such as making preparations to leave the house, with bags and buggy, whist saying 'Time to go shopping'). The informed observations of health visitors and nursery staff/child-minders can provide further corroboration of parental report.

In the home, nursery or clinic setting, the clinician has the opportunity both to observe communication between care-givers and child and to interact directly with the child. Key features to record include: the child's response to greetings, farewells and other social routines; joint referencing (looking to parents for reassurance and guidance); self-directed talk during play; functions of language directed to parents (showing and sharing, asking for help, giving information etc.); typical sentence length; speech intelligibility; and non-verbal communication.

BOX 5 Key stages in speech and language development

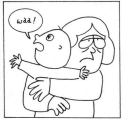

0–2 months
Discomfort cries

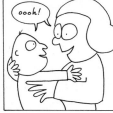

2–4 months
Pleasure sounds

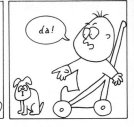

4–9 months
Babbling

9–12 months
Vocalisations with meaning

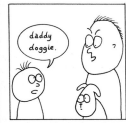

12–15 months
First words

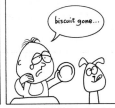

18–30 months
Word phrases

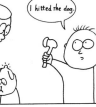

2½–4 years
Developing syntax

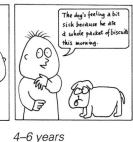

4–6 years
Adult syntax

Children may show delayed development in one or more areas of speech, language or communication development. Sensory deficits, neurological impairments of posture and movement execution or planning or a social impairment will all have significant implications for language learning. Alternatively, children may have specific language impairments. Assessment by a speech-and-language therapist will help to identify a child's strengths and difficulties, determine the need for multidisciplinary assessment and establish appropriate strategies to support communication development.

BOX 6 Bilingualism

On a world scale, monolingualism is unusual. Bilingualism, i.e., 'the knowledge and or use of two or more language codes . . . regardless of the relative proficiency of the languages understood or used' (RCSLT 2003) does not result in communication disorders. The limited research available suggests the same proporotion of bilingual and monolingual children will have speech and language disorders, and that any difficulties would occur in both languages and would be of a similar type, but that the errors made by the child may be language-specific (Holm et al. 2005).

Assessment of the communication skills of bilingual children and intervention for those with speech/language disorders is problematic due to limited knowledge about bilingual language development, a shortage of bilingual professionals and differing cultural views of language development and disorders. A thorough case history may provide some insight into parent's views about the presenting difficulties.

Language for learning

Children utilise their communication skills in the expression of needs and wants, to share information and interests, for the purposes of social closeness and for social etiquette. In addition, effective oral-language skills provide the basis for subsequent literacy and numeracy development. The impact of a communication delay or disability on reading and spelling is well recognised and one of the motivations for providing advice and support for parents in the early stage of development.

It has been estimated that up to 50 per cent of children in the UK start school lacking the communication skills necessary for an effective start to learning, most commonly in regions where there is socio-economic disadvantage (Locke et al. 2002). This delay is often specific to language, with the children having general cognitive skills comparable to the general population. Most of these children will have transient difficulties and are likely to catch up with their peers given appropriate support. Ten per cent of children can be described as having a communication disability (1.2 million in the UK), with 6 per cent having a specific and persistent communication disability (I CAN 2006).

Supporting language and communication development

Parents and other care-givers have a fundamental role in supporting communication development. General advice would be directed at enhancing the skills that most parents bring to interaction with the child.

Strategies to support communication

■ In the early months, talk to the baby, even when the baby is not talking back, particularly during care routines and play.

■ Respond to the baby's actions as if they have meaning.

■ Minimise background noise so babies can listen to speech.

■ Simplify speech: use short sentences, emphasise keywords, use gestures and leave pauses for the child to contribute.

■ Follow the child's attention and talk about what he/she is looking at for a short period on a daily basis.

■ Use everyday activities for language learning, e.g., putting away the shopping, sorting the laundry, etc.

■ Establish a daily routine of joint picture-book reading – talk about the pictures, rather than simply asking 'Where's the . . .?' or 'What's that?' questions.

All of these skills are used intuitively by parents and others who spend large amounts of time with young children. However, parents show variation in their levels of responsiveness and skill. Factors such as maternal depression, family stress and limited contact between children and parents may result in children receiving impoverished language input and are therefore important to explore during assessment.

Bochner, S., Price, P. and Jones, J. (1997) *Children's Language Development: Learning to Talk*. London: Whurr.

Buckley, B. (2003) *Children's Communication Skills: From Birth to Five Years*. London: Routledge.

Dockrell, J. and Messer, D. (1999) *Children's Language and Communication Difficulties: Understanding, Identification and Intervention*. London: Cassell.

Harris, M. (1992) *Language Experience and Early Language Development: From Input to Uptake*. Hove: LEA.

Further Reading

Social Behaviour and Play

Babies are born into a complex social world. Through active participation and guidance from people more skilled than themselves – adults and children, familiar and unfamiliar – children develop an understanding of the actions, intentions and feelings of others. This enables them to form and maintain relationships and to learn the conventions of behaviour within the society. From 2 months of age, parents and infants are able to hold each other's attention and engage in intricate, mutually regulated interchanges, primary intersubjectivity (Trevarthen and Aitken 2001). This 'dance' of social communication continues during infancy, with the baby learning social behaviour through familiar caregivers. The role of the caregivers changes as the child matures (see Table 6).

Table 6 Key stages in social development.

Age	Child's development	Roles of the caregiver
0–6 weeks	■ Preference for attending to people. ■ Recognition of mother's voice. ■ Intent regard of faces.	■ Treating infant as a communicating being. ■ Sympathetic and expressive behaviour that holds the infant's attention.
6–8 weeks	■ Smiling emerges. ■ Imitation of facial expressions.	■ Sustained interaction sequences, recognising the need for pauses and withdrawal to avoid over-excitement.
3 months	■ Smiling and other facial expressions synchronised with those of caregivers.	■ Developing social routines.
5 months	■ Growing interest in objects. ■ Some refusal to look at parents.	■ Developing games with objects in order to maintain interaction.
9 months	■ Using referential gaze to direct parent's attention to objects.	■ Following the infant's focus of attention.

10 months	■ Wary of strangers.	■ Offering reassurance – remaining close by. ■ Modelling friendly behaviour.	
1–2 years	■ Reactions to novel situations largely dependent on that of caregiver (social referencing). ■ Development of teasing – anticipating parent's reaction to forbidden actions. ■ Protest and tantrums – limit testing.	■ Modelling appropriate social behaviour. ■ Joint book reading – focusing on objects and actions. ■ Direct coaching – please, thank you, sorry, etc. ■ Setting standards and teaching permitted/forbidden behaviour.	
2–3 years	■ Understanding of responsibility – leading to denial of transgressions. ■ Asking 'what' and 'where' questions. ■ Captivated by stories – focus shifts from actions of characters to feelings.	■ Commenting and making suggestions during play. ■ Consistency in limit setting. ■ Direct coaching in polite behaviour. ■ Joint book reading – focusing on mental states.	
3–4 years	■ Breadth of interest in social world. ■ Asking 'why' questions. ■ Talk about inner states and rules – what is good, bad, naughty, allowed, etc. Able to adopt emotional states within pretend play.	■ Providing information and explanations of the actions of humans in social situations and stories.	
4–5 years	■ Growing understanding of rules. ■ Increasing understanding of the links between people's mental state and actions – theory of mind.	■ Supervision of games and play with peers. ■ Supporting social understanding.	

Play

Different types of play emerge as a child develops, assuming the conditions are supportive and materials are available. These stages are closely tied to cognitive, social and symbolic development (Table 7). Consequently, observation of play skills forms a crucial part of early years' assessment.

Development of play continues throughout the pre-school years, expressed variously in relation to age and developmental stage: for example, exploratory play in infancy includes mouthing toys; at 10 months the child may bang a cup on the table; at 2 years, he/she may climb into a box; at 4 years, he/she may be investigating bugs under stones in the garden.

Table 7 Cognitive and social sequences of play.

	Cognitive sequence	Social sequence
From birth	**Exploratory play** ■ Reflex activity. ■ Involuntary movements become purposeful through contingent responses, e.g., mobile moves when infant moves arm.	**Caregiver play** ■ Intent looking. ■ Imitation of facial expressions. ■ Vocalisations. ■ Actions become more purposeful through contingent responses.
5 months	**Coordinated orienting** ■ Visual regard and eye–hand coordination. ■ Exploration of objects – banging, mouthing.	**Integrated people–object play** ■ Toys can be the focus of shared attention – scaffolded by sensitive adult.
9 months	**Cause-and-effect play** ■ Targeted actions – pressing buttons, pulling strings – to obtain specific effects.	**Showing and sharing** ■ Holding up or offering toys in order to enlist adult in interaction.
12 months	**Functional play** ■ Use of common objects, e.g., putting on hat, 'talking' on phone.	
18 months	**Pretend play** ■ Using dolls as agents, e.g., feeding teddy.	**Joint interactive play with adults** ■ Taking turns with sensitive adult, e.g. ball play. ■ Imitating actions of adults.
2 years	**Play sequences** ■ Acting out familiar routines. **Symbolic play** ■ Use of placeholders, e.g., box as car.	**Parallel play** ■ Playing alongside other children.
3 years	**Imaginative play sequences** ■ Familiar activities and events. ■ Fantasy play.	**Associative play** ■ Sharing materials but pursuing own ideas.
4 years	**Narrative play** ■ Use of miniatures. ■ Creation of conventional and fantasy scenarios.	**Co-operative play** ■ Negotiation with peers. ■ Appreciation of rules.

The development of children's friendships provides a vehicle for, and a reflection of, increasing social understanding. From the age of 18 months, children demonstrate an increasing awareness of other children and respond in increasingly sophisticated ways, modifying their behaviour in the context of peer interaction (Table 8).

Development of friendships

Table 8 Stages in development of friendships.

18 months	■ Child shows awareness of another child's distress.
20 months	■ Mutual imitation. ■ Beginning to cooperate with a sibling/peer in order to achieve a goal.
2 years	■ Development of preferences for particular companions. ■ Cooperating within a shared play theme, e.g., a tea party.
2½ years	■ Able to adopt complementary roles within play scenarios, e.g., doctor–patient, mother–baby. ■ Awareness of what is pretence, e.g., pretending to be in pain, a hungry baby, etc.
3 years	■ Using references to friendship to include and exclude, e.g., 'I'm not your friend today'. ■ Tendency to label any play companion as a friend, therefore can appear fickle. ■ Development of 'fighting friends', i.e., reciprocal relationships that include both harmonious play and conflict. ■ Some children develop imaginary friends.
4 years	■ Children are clear about who their friends are and will differentiate between friends and other peers. ■ Development of sophisticated sharing of a pretend world. Play includes sustained adventures, often including favourite characters from books or films, or everyday events. ■ Fantasy play with strong emotional components such as fear, abandonment, bravery. ■ Alternative types of reciprocal play include sharing physical activities (chasing, playing football or skipping) or shared mischief.
5 years	■ Increasing understanding of the needs, feelings and wishes of friends. ■ Bargaining, compromise and reconciliation. ■ Able to talk about what makes someone a friend.

In early childhood, siblings often show a mix of concern and hostility towards one another. Teasing of parents and older siblings emerges from around 15 months, with children engaging in increasingly elaborate actions to annoy. There is evidence of strong attachments to older siblings from early in the second year. Siblings are generally able to cooperate to some degree in play by 3 years. By 4 years, children have developed the capacity to provide emotional support to distressed younger siblings.

Assessing play and social behaviour

Descriptions of behaviour in the home and other social settings can be obtained from parents. Direct observation can be made in the clinic if a range of play materials appropriate to age/developmental stage are available. In observing social behaviour, questions could include the following:

■ How does the child use the parent and other caregivers as a way of understanding and interacting with the world?

■ How does the child relate to siblings and peers?

■ Does the child show joint attention behaviours, showing and sharing, joint interactive play?

■ Is the child able to pretend? Pretending and speech emerge at around the same time and are closely related developmental skills.

■ Assessments such as the CHAT (Baron-Cohen et al. 1992) focus on early play, communication and social behaviours. Significant delay in social and behaviour and play can be associated with childhood autism (Baird et al. 2000).

Supporting social behaviour and play

Parents, caregivers and early years professionals play a crucial role in supporting a child's social development. The emphasis should be on creating opportunities rather than direct teaching of skills.

■ Creating distraction-free time for interaction with infants.

■ Creating opportunities for social play: action songs, turn-taking games, joint interactive play, joint book-reading.

■ Valuing children's play.

■ Providing age-appropriate play materials.

■ Sharing the excitement of children's discoveries and achievements.

- Supporting the development of peer relationships: taking turns, sharing, making requests, passing toys, etc.

- Direct coaching in polite behaviour.

- Consistent management of behaviour, with clear boundaries.

Further Reading

Carpendale, J. and Lewis, C. (2006) *How Children Develop Social Understanding.* Oxford: Blackwell.

Cohen, D. (2006) *The Development of Play*, 3rd edn. London: Routledge.

Dunn, J. (2003) *Children's Close Relationships: Beyond Attachment.* Oxford: Blackwell.

Dunn, J. (2004) *Children's Friendships: The Beginnings of Intimacy.* Oxford: Blackwell.

Harris, P. L. (2000) *The Work of the Imagination.* Oxford: Blackwell.

Sheridan, M. (1999) *Play in Early Childhood: From Birth to Six Years*, 2nd edn, rev. by J. Harding and L. Meldon-Smith. London: Routledge.

Attention, emotions and self-regulation

The development of self-regulation brings together strands from maturing attention, emotional regulation and planning and organising abilities (executive function). It is facilitated by the concurrently developing language, memory and improving processing ability or cognition and is influenced by emotional experience, attachment with care-givers and inherited temperament (Figure 7). In the early pre-school period, children begin to carry out intentional tasks or activities. They seem to have a plan when they pick up objects and toys. They start with simple activities such as stacking bricks, scribbling with a crayon, feeding themselves or a doll and, in time, move to more complex constructions, drawing and play sequences. To succeed in such planned and sequential activities, they must remember their plan in their working memory, organise their actions, overcome obstacles, manage their frustrations and emotions and ignore other distractions.

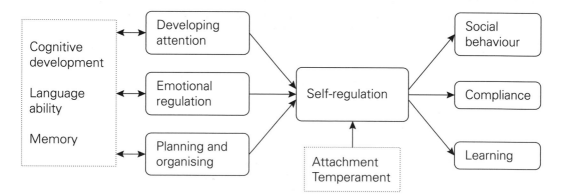

Figure 7 *Factors influencing self-regulation.*

Regulating emotions does not mean suppressing emotions but expressing emotions effectively and appropriately for getting one's needs met and for forming and maintaining social relationships. It has a crucial role for survival and socialisation. Infants express their needs and distress through crying and socialise by smiling. Over the next few years, children develop refined emotional understanding, expression and ways of regulating their emotions (Table 9). Within the first few months, infants show the ability to modulate their emotions by doing self-comforting activities such as sucking their thumb or seeking comfort from their carers. By 18 months, toddlers avoid or ignore emotionally arousing situations by talking to themselves or moving on to do something else. By 4 to 5 years, children know that they can hide their emotions or show a different emotion if need be. They begin to manage and control their emotions and become 'emotionally

Development of emotional awareness, expression and regulation

Table 9 Stages of emotional development.

	Emotional expression	Emotional awareness	Emotional regulation
Birth to four months	Crying Smiling Facial expression of distress, disgust, pleasure	Responds to maternal facial expressions	Self-soothing behaviour such as thumb sucking, body movements
5–6 months	Facial expression of anger	Responds to emotions in the face and voice of carers	
7–12 months	Displays wariness and fear to unfamiliar people Facial expressions of sadness (in response to maternal separation)	Social referencing – checking back – to carers' face and voice	Disengaging/avoiding attention
2–3 years	Displays shame and embarrassment Show empathy Uses emotion words	Able to decode and label others' emotions correctly	Information-seeking, e.g. social referencing
4–5 years	Expresses complex emotions Uses emotions to negotiate interactions with others.	Sophisticated understanding of causes and consequences of emotions	Hiding/modulating emotions and expressing socially appropriate emotions

self-sufficient'. However, it can still remain particularly challenging for children to deal with different expectations around how to express emotions at home and at school. The role of parents and carers changes from initially providing comfort and soothing to providing emotional support and to conveying social expectations for emotional expression. Children's ability to appropriately modulate their emotional expression is a combination of their own temperament and their learning from interactions with others.

Development of attention and self-organising ability

Within the first few weeks of birth, infants begin to turn towards faces, bright toys or interesting sounds. At this stage, their attention is brief and elicits a reflexive response. But, to remember and learn, infants must look or listen more than just briefly. This process of sustained or focused attention starts as early as the age of 3 months. Initially, the attention is sustained only for 5–10 seconds. By the age of 18 months, children have a good capacity to remain focused and interested long enough to begin to 'know' things. While paying attention, children look interested and calm. With further development, children need to spend less time looking at simple things and relatively longer at complex things or activities. When the mental effort becomes too much for their developmental ability, their attention is broken. Although children's ability to sustain attention improves with age, it remains a combination of their cognitive ability and their ability to control their impulsiveness and inhibit their distractibility towards other interests (Table 10).

By 4 years of age, children are able to sustain their attention to learn, plan a sequence of actions, inhibit their impulse to respond to interesting but irrelevant attractions and manage their emotions to stay on the task. They are now beginning to self-regulate their behaviour with gradually decreasing requirement for adults to guide and supervise their activities. Children mature in these abilities at different rates. Disruption in the development of self-regulation is one of the reasons for children to be disorganised, impulsive, defiant, easily frustrated and generally difficult. If such difficulties persist into early school years, a detailed assessment

Table 10 Stages of attention development.

Stage 1: First Year
　　　　High level of distractibility towards dominant stimuli

Stage 2: Second year
　　　　Rigid attention on a task of their own choice. Resistant to interference.

Stage 3: Third year (Single channelled attention)
　　　　Attention must be fully obtained to shift to a different task.

Stage 4: Fourth year (Early integrated attention)
　　　　Children can control their own focus of attention – need to look towards the carer to
　　　　listen.

Stage 5: Fifth year (Mature integrated attention)
　　　　Can perform an activity while listening to the carer/teacher giving directions.

Stage 6: Flexible and sustained attention

Based on Cooper, Moodley and Reynell (1978)

should be arranged to consider their general and language development, behaviour, attention, emotional and social well-being and other aspects of their health to include their hearing and vision (Richards 2005).

Children's ability to self-regulate their emotions and attention emerge in the context of care-giving relationships. Parents support the development of self-regulation through:

Supporting the development of self-regulation

■ providing predictable routines, through repeated patterns of asking and praising;

■ modelling behaviour;

■ direct coaching (e.g., asking the child to say sorry or comfort their friend or sibling or encouraging them to take turns);

■ gradually helping children to do things by themselves.

The praise and support that children get from their parents is an important resource for self-regulation. Some children need more support than others and for longer times. It can be a very different challenge for children with different temperaments or for children with a variety of diagnosed disabilities and for their care-givers. Advice may be available from local parenting support groups or child mental health services. There are some general skills and methods that parents can use to help their child's attention and self-regulation:

- Getting the child's attention:

    - Get the child to look at you in the eye, even by gently holding their hands and pointing their face towards yours.

    - Speak clearly, without shouting.

    - Turn off other distractions such as television/radio/music.

- Set up routines.

- Praise and be positive, reward the child for being good.

- Help the child to think before taking an action: set up a stop–think–act routine.

- Encourage children to talk about their feelings and experience after they have done something.

Further reading

Saarni, C. (1999) *The Development of Emotional Competence.* New York: Guilford.

Shonkoff, J. P. and Phillips, D. A. (eds) (2000) *From Neurons to Neighbourhood.* Washington, DC: National Research Council and Institute of Medicine/National Academy Press.

Sroufe, L. A. (1995) *Emotional Development: The Organization of Emotional Life in the Early Years.* Cambridge: Cambridge University Press.

Taylor, E. (ed.) (2007) *People with Hyperactivity: Understanding and Managing their Problem.* Clinics in Developmental Medicine 171. London: MacKeith Press.

Attachment and the development of self

Children's attachment is formed as a result of close affective relationship between the infant and the care-giver and is not simply a biological dependency. It has a stable organising role for social and emotional behaviours. The parent's sensitivity and motivation in reading the infant's signals and quality of their response forms the basis of the sense of security and trust for the infant. When the parent is not available or is unreliable, the infant feels less secure, and the infant's behaviour becomes less exploratory. A secure attachment relationship with the parent helps the infant form a stable working model of self and others (Bretherton and Waters 1985).

Attachment behaviours become increasingly differentiated with age (Table 11). Behaviours are also person- and context-dependent: e.g., in the home, they may show low-intensity behaviours such as smiling and approaching visitors; in other situations they may show high-intensity behaviours such as wanting to be picked up or stay close to their primary care-givers.

Development of attachment behaviour

Table 11 Attachment characteristics.

	Orientation towards a care-giver
Birth onwards	Preferential orientation towards one person
5 months onwards	Proximity-seeking and separation protest
7 to 9 months onwards	Able to wait if a reason is explained
Third and fourth year	Able to understand care-giver's plan or motivation.
Fourth year onwards	Relationship based on abstract considerations such as affection and trust.

As children grow, a number of factors affect their attachment behaviours (Box 7). As children reach school age, their social world expands to include other relationships, attachment becomes less dependent on literal and more on symbolic proximity, and they can tolerate longer periods of separation. There is often a reversal to earlier stages during periods of distress.

> **BOX 7** Factors influencing attachment behaviours
>
> ■ Developing cognitive understanding such as 'object permanence' (the mother who has left the room is still around) and reasoning (understanding explanations).
>
> ■ Improving communication skills.
>
> ■ Development of 'social referencing' (need to check or show) and perspective taking.
>
> ■ Experience of periods of separation.
>
> ■ Better coping skills.
>
> ■ Family and cultural routines.

Patterns of attachment

Ainsworth, based on a Strange Situation Test, described distinct patterns of infants' behaviour to indicate the quality of their attachment with their parents (Ainsworth et al. 1978).

■ Securely attached infants show a high quality, relatively unambivalent relationship with the care-giver. They may be upset when the care-giver leaves, are happy to see the care-giver return and recover quickly from any distress.

■ Insecurely attached infants have a less positive attachment to their care-givers and are described as being either:

■ **Insecure/resistant**: Infants or young children are clingy, stay close to the care-giver, get very upset when the care-giver leaves and are not comforted by strangers. They are not easily comforted and both seek comfort and resist efforts by the care-givers to comfort them.

- **Insecure/avoidant**: Infants or young children seem indifferent toward their care-giver and may even avoid the care-giver. If they get upset alone they are comforted as easily by a stranger as by a parent.

- **Disorganised/disoriented**: Infants or young children have no consistent way of coping with the situation of being left alone with a stranger. Their behaviour is often confused or even contradictory, and they often appear disoriented (Main and Soloman 1986).

Secure infants are able to use their mother as a base to explore, are related to sensitive and consistent parenting and have a generally better social and psychological functioning in later life than insecure infants.

Interpreting attachment behaviours

A simplistic interpretation of children's attachment behaviours can do more harm than good through misattribution of causal links or consequences. Children's attachment behaviours are influenced by their developmental abilities and a number of other behaviour systems such as exploratory behaviour, stranger awareness, social or affiliative behaviour, fear/anxiety and temperament. Strong or weak attachment behaviours do not necessarily represent strong or weak attachments. Children show strong or weak attachment behaviours depending on intensity or the strength of the situation in which these are activated and not on how well or poorly they are attached to the person. A securely attached child may greet the mother by running up to her and hugging her in one situation and by smiling and waving in another. The strength of the attachment with a care-giver depends on the history of relationship with that care-giver and is reflected in the level of security it provides to the child.

The development of self

A developing sense of self as an individual is important because the way individuals view themselves appears to influence the overall feelings of well-being and competence. The sense of self emerges early in infancy and is an ongoing and complex process. By 4 to 5 months of age, infants express themselves through anger. From 9 to 12 months of age, infants begin to show joint attention with others to share their interests, indicating that they have a sense of separation from others. Their emerging recognition of the self becomes clearer by 18–20 months of age when they recognise their image in a mirror as themselves; and when they notice a dot or colour on their face, they try to remove it from their face and not from the mirror – as they would have done earlier, indicating that they realise that the mirror image is a self-reflection. By the age of 2 years, they begin to pick themselves out from pictures, show emotions of embarrassment and shame and begin to self-assert themselves through temper tantrums. By 3–4 years, children understand themselves in terms of concrete, observable characteristics related to physical attributes and their relationships. In the pre-school years, children tend to think they are as they wish to be, such as being good at something. In the coming years, they begin the process of comparing themselves with others.

Supporting self-esteem

Parents contribute to the child's developing self-image by giving criticism or praise and positive or negative descriptions of their behaviour and by reminding them of their successes or failures. This influences children's perceptions of themselves, which, in turn, plays a role in how they respond to their successes and failures. Some children, when they face a difficulty or a failure, blame themselves and stop trying whilst others persevere. Children who are supported in verbalising, analysing and describing their negative beliefs about themselves, given opportunities to succeed and praised for achieving success, have fewer problem behaviours and a better sense of self-esteem.

Further reading

Damon, W. and Hart, D. (1988) *Self-Understanding in Childhood and Adolescence*. Cambridge: Cambridge University Press.
Parkes, C. M., Stevenson-Hinde, J. and Marris, P. (1996) *Attachment across the Lifecycle*. London: Routledge.

Hearing

Awareness of children's hearing behaviour forms the basis for eliciting parental concerns and behavioural tests of hearing. At birth, infants show a preference for their mother's speech, likely to be based on their well-established ability to hear from about 3 months before birth. Newborns are able to discriminate between the general direction of a sound (left or right, far or near), but orienting towards more subtle variations in location improves over the next 6 months. Infants can discriminate vowels after birth; by 2–3 months they can discriminate the fine differences between phonemes such as /da/, /ba/ and /pa/, and by 6 months their speech discrimination is well refined. In some aspects, infants' speech perception is superior to that of adults, and before 6 months of age, they can discriminate speech sounds in their own and in other languages. By 10–12 months, however, infant sound perception becomes much more adult-like, with reduced perception of sounds in other languages. Children growing up in bilingual families, however, maintain their ability for sound discrimination for the languages used.

Development of hearing behaviour

Significant sensorineural hearing loss (SNHL), requiring a hearing aid, is present in about 16 per 10,000 children. Conductive hearing loss is extremely common. At least half of pre-school children have one or more episodes of 'glue ear', or otitis media with effusion (OME). Persistent OME, which may have adverse effects on children's language and behaviour, affects about 5–10 per cent of children. Parental smoking is a risk factor for children developing OME (see Box 8).

Hearing impairment

Early identification

Delayed identification of children with congenital or acquired hearing loss may result in deficits in speech and language development, poor educational achievement and behaviour and emotional difficulties. Early identification of hearing loss and appropriate intervention has been shown to prevent many of these adverse consequences. The main strategies for early identification include:

- screening for hearing defects;

- recognising children who are at risk for congenital or acquired hearing loss (Box 8) or have conditions associated with hearing loss, such as language or general developmental delay;

- eliciting concerns (Appendix 1) and promptly responding to parental concerns. (Parents often report suspicion of hearing loss, inattention or erratic response to sound before hearing loss is confirmed.);

- hearing assessment of those with risks and concerns (Table 12).

A thorough general examination is an essential part of evaluation of a child with hearing loss. Findings associated with hearing impairment include heterochromia of the irises, malformation of the auricle or ear canal, dimpling or skin tags around the auricle, cleft lip or palate, asymmetry or hypoplasia of the facial structures, microcephaly and abnormal pigmentation of hair or skin.

Table 12 Audiological tests for infants and children.

Physiological tests	■ Evoked or automated otoacoustic emissions (OAE) ■ Automated brainstem responses (ABR) These tests measure cochlear/brainstem responses to sounds.
Behavioural tests 7–18 months	■ Distraction hearing test ■ Visually reinforced audiometry Developmental age of 7 months is optimum for the distraction test. A soundproof environment and trained testers are essential.
2–4 years	■ Play audiometry Child attention span may limit the success of the test.
3.5 years onwards	■ Conventional audiometry Speech and frequency-specific stimuli presented through earphones.

Vision

Development of visual behaviour

Awareness of the development of normal visual behaviour helps in identifying vision defects. These may be severe, though treatable, or may require early developmental guidance. Developmental visual behaviours during early childhood (Table 13) provide a basis for eliciting concerns from parents (Appendix 2) and for making observations to identify children in need of further specialist examination. However, these are not tests for vision and can seriously underestimate the severity of any vision defect.

Table 13 Stages of development of visual behaviour.

Birth	Turns eyes towards window or any large light source.
First month	Stares at object close to their face and shows special interest in human face.
4 to 6 weeks	Defensive blink is present.
3 months	Watches own hands. Follows activities in the surroundings.
6 months	Looks intently on a 2.5 centimetre brick at 30 centimetres. Recognises carers and familiar toys from across the room.
9 months	Looks intently at small objects up to 1 millimetre in size (e.g., crumbs or 'hundreds and thousands' cake decorations) and uses fingers to poke. Points to demand nearby objects.
12 months	Points to show objects of interest at a distance.

Sustained poor visual fixation, abnormal or wandering eye movements and a squint or a 'lazy eye' may indicate the presence of a visual defect at any age.

Poor visual behaviour or presence of squint or abnormal eye movements can be presenting features of a rare but serious eye condition or systemic disorders such as a cataract, glaucoma and retinoblastoma, which are sight or life-threatening and are treatable. The most common vision disorders among children are squint, amblyopia and optical problems impairing visual acuity. At least 2 per cent of children have amblyopia, a condition of reduced vision in which the eye itself is healthy, but because of a difference between vision in each eye or squint the brain has either suppressed or failed to develop the visual function. It is usually unilateral but rarely may be bilateral. About 1 per cent of infants and 3–7 per cent of young children have a squint.

Vision impairment

A combination of a proactive examination of all children's eyes and vision, observation of visual behaviour of children presenting with neuro-developmental problems and eliciting and promptly responding to parental concerns provides a good basis for early identification of visual impairments (Box 9). Children with poor vision require specialist examination of eyes, developmental guidance and early educational advice by specialist teachers.

Early identification

> **BOX 9** Surveillance of vision
>
> ■ An ophthalmoscopic examination of eye of all newborns to look for red reflex, repeated at 6–8 weeks, is essential to exclude serious conditions such as congenital cataract and retinoblastoma.
>
> ■ Infants who are born prematurely or with a family history of heritable eye disorders should have specialist examination by an ophthalmologist.
>
> ■ Children whose parents are concerned about their vision, or have poor visual behaviour, squint or abnormal eye movements should have an orthoptic examination.

- Formal tests for visual acuity in pre-school children are best carried out by orthoptists. The Sonksen Silver test for visual acuity can be used from age 3 years and older children. Each eye must be tested separately, with the other eye occluded.

- The majority of squints are first recognised by parents. Some squints are not apparent on simple inspection and the cover–uncover test or the alternate cover test may be used. The performance and interpretation of these tests is not easy and orthoptic assessment should be arranged in case of doubt and when there are parental concerns or relevant family history.

Checklist for detection of hearing problems

Hint for parents

Can your baby hear you?

Here is a checklist of some of the general signs you can look for in your baby's first year (with acknowledgements to Dr Barry McCormick). Does your baby display the following characteristics?

YES/NO

Shortly after birth
Your baby should be startled by a sudden loud noise such as a hand clap or a door slamming, and should blink or open her/his eyes widely to such sounds.

By 1 month
Your baby should be beginning to notice sudden or prolonged sounds like the noise of a vacuum cleaner and s/he should pause and listen to them when they begin.

By 4 months
S/he should quieten or smile at the sound of your voice when s/he cannot see you. S/he may also turn her/his head or eyes towards you if you come up from behind and speak to her/him from the side.

By 7 months
S/he should turn immediately to your voice from across the room or to very quiet noises on each side if s/he is not too occupied with other things.

By 9 months
S/he should listen attentively to familiar everyday sounds and search for very quiet sounds made out of sight. S/he should also show pleasure in babbling loudly and tunefully.

By 12 months
S/he should show some response to her/his own name and to other familiar words. S/he may also respond when you say 'no' and 'bye-bye', even when s/he cannot see any accompanying gesture.

Your health visitor will perform a routine hearing test on your baby between six and eight months of age. She will be able to help and advise you at any time before or after this test if you are concerned about your baby and her/his development. If you suspect that your baby is not hearing normally, either because you cannot answer 'yes' to the items above or for some other reason, seek advice from your health visitor.

© Dr Barry McCormick, Children's Hearing Assessment Centre, Nottingham

Appendix 2 | Checklist for detection of vision problems

Here are some of the signs of normal vision for you to look out for during your baby's first year:

From 1 week

- ■ Does your baby turn to diffuse light?
- ■ Does your baby stare at your face?

By 2 months

- ■ Does your baby look at you, follow your face if you move from side to side, and smile responsively back at you?
- ■ Do your baby's eyes move together?

By 6 months

- ■ Does your baby look around with interest?
- ■ Does your baby try to reach out for small objects?
- ■ Do you think your baby has a squint? (Squint is now definitely abnormal, however slight and temporary.)

By 9 months

- ■ Does your baby poke and rake very small objects such as crumbs or 'hundreds and thousands' cake decorations with fingers?

By 12 months

- ■ Does your baby point to things to demand?
- ■ Does your baby recognise people he/she knows from across the room, before they speak to him/her?

> **If at any time you suspect that your baby's vision is not normal, either because you cannot answer 'Yes' to any of the items above or you suspect a squint, seek advice from your health visitor or general practitioner.**

Internet-based Resources

www.afasic.org.uk

Afasic is a UK charity which supports children and young people with speech, language and communication impairments and their parents and carers. Information on language development and disorders and how to get help.

www.ican.org.uk

I CAN is a UK charity aiming to support the development of all children's speech, language and communication, focusing particularly on those with communication disorders. Provider of information and direct services.

Resources include free DVDs:

- *Chatter Matters*: advice for parents on supporting language development.
- *Learning to Talk*: for early years professionals.

www.literacytrust.org.uk/talktoyourbaby

A campaign run by the National Literacy Trust to encourage parents and carers to talk more to children from birth to 3 years. Useful information sheets on early communication and on development of reading and writing. Also resources on attachment.

www.childrensproject.co.uk

The Children's Project is a source of books and materials for parents with young families and professionals supporting and promoting early years development.

www.surestart.gov.uk

A Government programme providing information on early education, child care, health and family support. Links to *From Birth to Three Matters* – information for child-care professionals on child development, effective practice, examples of play activities to promote play/learning, guidance on planning/resources and meeting diverse needs.

www.nlm.nih.gov/medlineplus/childdevelopment.html#cat1 and www.cdc.gov/ncbddd/child

US websites for information on overview, initiatives and information regarding child development.

www.everychildmatters.gov.uk

Every Child Matters proposed the introduction of a national common assessment framework as an important part of a strategy for helping children.

www.everychildmatters.gov.uk/deliveringservices/ commoncore/development

Describes the common core skills and knowledge in relation to child development for professionals working with children.

www.earlysupport.org.uk and www.cafamily.org.uk

Information and resources for children with disabilities and special needs.

References

Ainsworth, M. D. S., Blehar, M., Waters, S. E. and Wall, S. (1978) *Patterns of Attachment: A Psychological Study of the Strange Situation*. Hillsdale, NJ: Erlbaum.

Amiel-Tison C. and Grenier A. (1986) *Neurological Assessment during the First Year of Life*. Oxford: Oxford University Press.

Baird G., Charman, T., Baron-Cohen, S., Cox, A., Swettenham, J., Wheelwright, S., Drew, A. (2000) 'A Screening Instrument for Autism at 18 Months of Age: A 6-Year Follow-Up Study', *Journal of the American Academy of Child and Adolescent Psychiatry* 39 (6): 694–702.

Baron-Cohen, S., Allen, J., Gillberg, C. (1992) 'Can Autism be Detected at 18 Months? The Needles, the Haystack, and the CHAT', *British Journal of Psychiatry* 161 (December): 839–43.

Bly, L. (1994) *Motor Skills Acquisition in the First year: An Illustrated Guide to Normal Development*. Tucson, Ariz.: Therapy Skill Builders.

Brazelton, T. B. and Nugent, J. K. (1995) *The Neonatal Behavioral Assessment Scale*. Cambridge: MacKeith Press.

Bretherton, I. and Waters, E. (1985) *Growing Points of Attachment Theory and Research*. Chicago, Ill.: University of Chicago Press for the Society for Research in Child Development.

Bruner, J. (1983) *Child's Talk: Learning to Use Language*. New York: W. W. Norton.

Bzoch, M. and League, R. (1991) *Receptive-Expressive Emergent Language Scales*, 2nd edn. Austin, Tex.: PRO-ED Inc.

Cooper, J., Moodley, M. and Reynell, J. (1978) *Helping Language Development: A Developmental Programme for Children with Early Learning Handicaps*. London: Edward Arnold.

Fenson, L., Dale, P. S., Reznick, J. S., Thal, D., Bates, E., Hartung, J. P., Pethick, S. and Reilly, J. S. (1993) *MacArthur Communicative Development Inventory: User's Guide and Technical Manual*. Baltimore, Md.: Paul H. Brookes.

Frankenburg, W. K., Dodds, J. B., Fandal, A. W., Kazuk, E. and Cohrs, M. (1975) *The Denver Developmental Screening Test*. Denver, Col.: University of Colorado Medical Centre.

Galluhe, D. I. and Ozmum, J. C. (2006) *Understanding Motor Development*, 6th edn. New York: McGraw-Hill.

Holm, A., Stow, C. and Dodd, B. (2005) 'Bilingual Children with Phonological Disorders: Identification and Intervention', in B. Dodd (ed.), *Differential Diagnosis and Treatment of Children with Speech Disorder*, 2nd edn. London: Whurr, pp. 275–88.

I CAN (2006) *The Cost to the Nation of Children's Poor Communication*. London: I CAN.

Locke, A., Ginsborg, J. and Peers, I. (2002) 'Development and Disadvantage: Implications for the Early Years and Beyond', *International Journal of Language and Communication Disorders* 37 (1): 3–16.

Main, M. and Soloman, J. (1986) 'Discovery of an Insecure Disorganized/Disorientated Attachment Pattern: Procedures, Findings and Implications for the Classification of Behaviour', in T. B. Brazelton and M. Yogman (eds), *Affective Development in Infancy*. Norwood, NJ: Ablex.

Milani-Comparetti, A. and Gidoni, E. A. (1967) 'Routine Developmental Examination in Normal and Retarded Children', *Developmental Medicine and Child Neurology* 9 (9): 631–8.

Newson, J. (1979) 'The Growth of Shared Understandings between Infant and Caregiver', in C. Bullowa (ed.), *Before Speech*. Cambridge: Cambridge University Press, pp. 207–22.

Piek, J. P. (2006) *Infant Motor Development*. Champaign, Ill: Human Kinetics.

Prechtl, H. F. R. (1977) *The Neurological Examination of the Fullterm Newborn Infant*, 2nd edn. Clinics in Developmental Medicine 63. London: McKeith Press.

RCSLT (2003) *Core Guidelines*. London: RCSLT

Reddy, V., Hay, D., Murray, L. and Trevarthen, C. (1997) 'Communication in Infancy: Mutual Regulation of Affect and Attention', in G. Bremner, A. Slater and G. Butterworth (eds), *Infant Development: Recent Advances*. Hove: Psychology Press, pp. 247–74.

Richards, J. E. (2005) 'Attention', in B. Hopkins (ed.), *The Cambridge Encyclopedia of Child Development*, Cambridge: Cambridge University Press, pp. 282–6.

Robson, P. (1984) 'Prewalking Locomotor Movements and their Use in Predicting Standing and Walking', *Child Care Health and Development* 10 (5): 317–30.

Sroufe, L. A. (1983) 'Patterns of Individual Adaptation from Infancy to Preschool: The Roots of Maladaptation and Competence', in M. Perlmutter (ed.), *Minnesota Symposia on Child Psychology* 16. Hillsdale, NJ: Lawrence Erlbaum, pp. 41–3.

Thelen, E. (1995) 'Motor Development: A New Synthesis', *American Psychologist* 50 (2): 79–95.

Tomasello, M. (1995) 'Joint Attention as Social Cognition', in C. Moore and P. J. Dunham (eds), *Joint Attention: Its Origins and Role in Development Symposia on Child Psychology*. Hillsdale, NJ: Lawrence Erlbaum Associates, pp. 41–83.

Trevarthen, C. and Aitken, K. J. (2001) 'Infant Intersubjectivity: Research, Theory, and Clinical Applications', *Journal of Child Psychology and Psychiatry*, 42 (1): 3–48.